Here is a self-help aid as simple as an Aesop Fable or the little train that said, "I think I can, I think I can . . . ." It is the Billfold Booster that has caught the fancy of the world and reminded many that they can change their lives by changing their attitudes of mind. The charts have been translated into many languages such as Japanese, Russian, Spanish, German, Norwegian, French and even set in Braille for the sightless.

The folders focus on thoughts and attitudes, the paths to spirituality, and have been used by all ages and all types of groups such as these . . . . .

Congressional prayer meetings in Washington, D.C.

A self-help group in Russia

Teen-age groups in Hawaii

Four thousand employees of Tokyo Telephone Co.

Prison inmates in Texas

A football team that won the Rose Bowl

A tulip farm in Holland

A doctor's clinic in Australia

The list goes on and on—churches, schools, armed forces, hospitals, retreat centers, sales conventions, social service agencies, governmental agencies, and corporations the world over have touched the lives of millions with the "boosters".

You are invited to share the enclosed Billfold Boosters with others. Many churches and hospitals have done this by placing the enclosed placard on a table with a supply of the folders beside it.

If you need more write to Clifftop Publishing Co., P.O. Box 44847, Eden Prairie, MN 55344. No charge for any reasonable number.

"Wholeness is not something that is created; it is a state of awareness. It is becoming awake to the co-existence of all the inner parts of life. What does it mean to be whole? Being whole is to become fully alive," says Robert Conklin in his new and wonderful book of empowerment, *Be Whole!* As I read each chapter I was frankly awed by the sense, insight, spirituality and validity of Mr. Conklin's message. His words flowed like a river of right and the overall effect brought me a glorious feeling that this is a direction to a path of betterment. *Be Whole!* does what great books do…it gets you to think. In this case, Robert Conklin not only gets you to think…he gets you to think about a message that is surely empowering.

Richard Fuller, Syndicated Columnist

An old proverb assures us that when the student is ready the teacher will appear. Robert Conklin is a masterful teacher as *Be Whole!* wisely and warmly illustrates. If you're ready for the joy, abundance and serenity that are the gifts of wholeness, make this book the next stop on your spiritual journey.

Barbara J. Winter
Author, *Making a Living Without a Job*

What a wealth of inspirational thoughts to help the reader *Be Whole!*…a fresh view all in the frame of "What you are taught can bind you; what you learn can free you. Learn to learn. Escape from self-inflicted restrictions." The rich inclusion of incidents, examples from everyday lives, illustrations from participants in your programs and reflections of personal testimony convincingly document the validity of people to *Be Whole!* My Life Coach, my own personal life trainer is available to me in this book. Thanks for providing me my own personal life trainer that is at my fingertips in the form of *Be Whole!* This source will be at the top of the recommended reading list!

Harriet B. Stephenson, Ph.D.
Professor of Management/Seattle University
Director, The Entrepreneurship Center

Robert Conklin has come up with new concepts and ideas in *Be Whole!* It is truly a wonderful piece of work by the author of the best personal growth program in the world—*Adventures in Attitudes!*

Dr. Dean Nelson
Psychologist/Human Resources Consultant

BE Whole!

Robert Conklin

Printed in the United States of America.

J I H G F E D C B A

First Edition 1997

Library of Congress Catalog Card Number 96-92796

ISBN 0-9654882-0-9

DISTRIBUTED TO THE TRADE BY:
LPC Group
1436 West Randolph Street
Chicago, IL 60607
(800) 626-4330

Dedicated...

*...to you, the reader. Without you
this book would not have been written.*

Also by Robert Conklin:

Think Yourself To The Riches of Life
The Power Of A Magnetic Personality
How To Get People To Do Things
The Dynamics of Successful Attitudes
EgoBionics

Thirty Hour Personal Development Programs:

Adventures in Attitudes
Life Power

Five Hour Attitude Assessment Program:

The Positive Mind

Contents

Prologue

DR. RENN, MY FRIEND, SPOKE SOFTLY AND SERIOUSLY. "I have gone over all the examination results very carefully. Frankly, I don't know how you had the strength to come in here. You want me to be honest with you. So I must tell you. I believe you have only a few weeks to live, six at the most."

But then they began—miracle after miracle. My life was saved so that I might help others save theirs.

Saving a life does not always mean avoiding death. It may mean rising above sickness, adversity, or despair, and finding wholeness, success, and love. Those who do so are empowered. By intent or intuition they uncover certain inner passages to personal empowerment.

Such an endowment can be learned. For life is a school. There are lessons, assignments, and tests. And grades for which one is personally responsible. Teachers, often unrecognized, are available. But they do not do the lessons and assignments. They only tutor and enlighten.

If the lessons are learned, the assignments completed, and the tests of life are met, then one can go on to the next level. Otherwise the lessons are repeated until they are learned.

This is a book about one course in life—personal empowerment and wholeness. There are lessons. And assignments—eight, in fact. Work on the assignments and you will become empowered. You will be whole. Miracles will happen along the way. Life will be better. I promise.

❧ THE EIGHT ASSIGNMENTS ❧

1. Surrender and connect.

2. Be miracle-minded.

3. Build positive attitudes.

4. Love unconditionally.

5. To the degree you give others what they need, they will give you what you need.

6. Visualize! Verbalize! Vitalize!

7. Learn to learn.

8. Reach for the sun.

ONE

In Search of Wholeness

> *"...be of good comfort; thy faith*
> *hath made thee whole."*
> —*Matthew 9:22*

WHAT DOES IT MEAN TO BE WHOLE?

Wholeness is not something that is created; it is a state of awareness. It is becoming awake to the co-existence of all the inner parts of life.

The people asked the Buddha, "Are you a God?"

"No," answered the Buddha.

"Are you an angel?"

"No."

"Then what are you?"

"I am awake."

The desire for awakening is the prelude to understanding wholeness. The search for wholeness is to know that you are already there. God made you whole. Eons were spent doing that. Every breath, every thought, every mood, every feeling, every cell of your body is a gift of God given to you for a purpose.

You can distort your wholeness. There seems to be a mortal urge to reinvent the human being. With scalpel thinking we divide ourselves into parts. Then with the same scalpel we tend to carve out that which, in our judgment or others' judgment, is a distasteful part of our nature. Inner strife results, one part against another. Our wholeness becomes fragmented. There is no peace, no comfort, no tranquility.

Completely overlooked is the nature of our wholeness. We are each a center of the universe; a universal wholeness extends out from our centers to infinity. We are all microcosms of the universe—a universe composed of diversities.

There are stormy days and quiet days, sunny days and cloudy days, warm temperatures and cold temperatures, deserts and oceans, stars and moons, cyclones, lightning, wind, rain, and drought—all diversities functioning in divine order in perfect harmony, balance, and synergy. That's wholeness.

As people are microcosms of the universe, the same diversities exist within us, within you. You are a sum total of your parts— many paths—emotional, physical, mental, and spiritual. Those have been cloned by an assortment of experiences, many joyful and enriching. But, perhaps, there have been disturbing influences— soured relationships, emotional pain, sickness, grief, suffering, lost promotions, family problems, worry, dreams that never happened, misplaced trust, loneliness—all of which are parts of your wholeness.

At the center of all your parts is a soul—a core of wholeness. Love is the bond that holds all parts together. Love yourself. Not the fragmented self, but the whole self—the miraculous, magnificient self, the center of the universe self.

My greatest wish for you is that you like yourself, love yourself, bless yourself, forgive yourself for all of the negative thoughts you have impressed into your mind and body that affect your wholeness.

What does it mean to be whole?

Being whole is to become fully alive.

It is enabling you to live life where it is happening—the present moment. The only life that you can experience is now, not trying to go back to the fleeting comfort of a yesterday. Nor is life something that will happen on the next vacation or when the bills are paid or when the right person comes along.

Wholeness means finding joy, purpose and satisfaction in this very moment, in every event, even those that may cause transient spaces of anguish or frustration.

Wholeness is to know that there is no condition in your life that cannot be healed, whether it be sickness, grief, chaos, poverty, or ruptured relationships. Life is ordained by your creative source to be good and you have the power to attract that.

Wholeness is looking within and finding resources and qualities that have eluded your awareness. It is to give you the courage to travel the unknown, to wander within the abyss of your soul seeking the rewards of a limitless life beyond that which you have known.

Wholeness is to deepen your capacity to enjoy work, family, friends, and your own individuality. It is the ability to sort out relationships nourishing those that satisfy your hunger for oneness. It is to be strengthened rather than weakened by people and circumstances.

Wholeness is to exist lovingly and harmoniously within the circumference of human nature, yours and others, rather than struggling to get outside that circle into the illusions of perfection—the perfect child, the perfect mate, the perfect lover, the perfect job. Wholeness recognizes that you live in an imperfect world of imperfect people. The only perfection that you can ever seek is the spiritual nature that rests within. To pursue that perfection is to glorify your wholeness.

Whoever you are, however you feel about yourself, no matter what you are facing, you are whole. Know that. Believe that and "thy faith hath made thee whole."

Do not blame, criticize, condemn or degrade yourself. Do not discard or repress your feelings or individuality. How can you become whole when stressed out by berating, denouncing, and badgering increments of your humanness? Quiet the battle within. God did not create only a part of you, but all of you—the spiritual, emotional, mental, physical—every cell, every organ, every facet of your mortality is an idea of your Creator. Wholeness is achieved by integrating, synchronizing, and harmonizing all parts of you into a synergistic whole. That's getting in touch with your soul, your spirit.

That is also personal empowerment. Wholeness is a state of being; personal empowerment is acquired. Personal empowerment respects your wholeness.

BE EMPOWERED! BE WHOLE!

Personal empowerment is the custodian of your wholeness.

Wholeness is the blossom of the soul. Knowing and caring for that blossom asks for personal empowerment.

Wholeness is a state of being authenticating your humanness. Empowerment is learned, developed, acquired.

Empowerment is a spiritual quest making holy your wholeness. Empowerment is the mobilization of your inner resources to maintain and strengthen your wholeness. Being empowered is to be in control of your mind, emotions, and behavior.

By being empowered, you maintain and enhance your wholeness, protecting it against cynicism, distress and all the other insidious influences that try to creep in and contaminate your wholeness.

Wholeness is like the sculptor's clay—soft and pliable. Personal empowerment is the artistry that molds the clay into beauty and symmetry.

So personal empowerment provides the tools by which you manage your wholeness.

EMPOWERMENT SHAPES WHOLENESS

To face adversity or setbacks with candor and honesty is wholeness; to convert those situations into opportunities is empowerment.

To have an appetite for food is wholeness; to eat wisely is empowerment.

To know the sorrows and pains as well as the joy and ecstasies of love is wholeness; to experience love as the spirit of God living in and through all life is empowerment.

To know that there are fears and doubts holding one back is wholeness; to be free of those is empowerment.

To recognize a desire for worldly things and pleasures is wholeness; to temper those desires with discipline and rationality is empowerment.

To feel anger is wholeness; to transform the energy of that anger into constructive behavior is empowerment.

To sense sexual desires without repression or guilt is wholeness; to find expressions for those feelings beautifully and lovingly is empowerment.

To feel inferior, inadequate, or belittled is wholeness; to transcend those feelings with self-assurance and self-esteem is empowerment.

To become aware of the limitations or impairments of the physical body by sickness or injury is wholeness; to refuse to allow such conditions to detract from the endearment of life is empowerment.

To experience fear is wholeness; to avoid being restrained or mastered by fear is empowerment.

To allow the ego to handle the practical circumstances of life is wholeness; to saturate the ego with the soul is empowerment.

To feel overwhelmed with undone tasks is wholeness; to value doing nothing when there is something to do is empowerment.

To acknowledge hate is wholeness; to dilute such feelings with understanding and love is empowerment.

To experience rejection and unfair treatment by others is wholeness; to refrain from criticism, revenge, or blame is empowerment.

To confess to guilt is wholeness; to stop doing or being what causes guilt is empowerment.

To admit to mistakes and failures is wholeness; to transform them into lessons of life is empowerment.

To feel voids of a spiritual presence or isolated from a higher power is wholeness; for such notions to stimulate the spiritual quest is empowerment.

To look beneath the surface texture of the mind and find pools of distress or despair is wholeness; to drain those off with patience and hope is empowerment.

To become aware of the ego's impulsive demands is wholeness; to guide such forces toward higher and more usable deeds of service is empowerment.

To revel in one's blessedness and good fortune is wholeness; to share that with others is empowerment.

To find dark and ominous thoughts hidden in the mind is wholeness; to know that such thoughts are merely reminders to be constantly cleansing and purifying the mind is empowerment.

To find life sometimes repetitious and burdensome is wholeness; to maintain a passion for living is empowerment.

To do nothing but sit and watch a spider spin a web, to feel the sunshine warm the air, or envision cloud pictures in the sky acccepting the nothingness of the moment in place of something-ness is wholeness; to find meaning and richness in such spaces is empowerment.

YOU WILL LEARN TO BE EMPOWERED

The key to wholeness is personal empowerment. Personal empowerment nourishes, shapes, and sustains your wholeness. The increments of your wholeness—mind, body, soul, spirit—will flourish and be strengthened by personal empowerment.

The purpose and emphasis of this book is to give you specific steps and instructions for enhancing your personal empowerment. Empowerment is learned and developed by wrestling with life's deeper, richer, and more significant meanings.

As with any learning experience, there are lessons. In fact, every encounter with another, every event, every circumstance, no matter how trivial, is a lesson. Lessons will be repeated until they are learned. When a lesson is learned you can then go on to the next one.

There are tests. At times the tests may be difficult. They may cause sorrow, struggle, pain, or distress. Know, however, that there is no test that cannot be passed. Inner strength and resources will always be found if earnestly sought. By meeting and going through any of the tests of life, additional sinews of personal empowerment are gained.

The essence of any learning and growth process are the assignments—studies and exercises. So it is with personal empowerment. There are eight assignments, projects of self-discovery and personal development. Each one, practiced with diligence, will be a powerful life-long tool for strengthening personal empowerment. Your resolve and determination will be reflected in the value you receive in each assignment.

At the beginning of a school year, the teacher always starts with an orientation talk. I still remember the one given when I entered college. The head of the university spoke about dedication, perseverance, studying, working to get the most out of education. Imprinted in my impressionable mind was: "The value of your experience here will be determined by the temperature of your desire."

That brings us to the next chapter, which is, really, an orientation presentation before you begin the eight assignments. Like the head of the university, the chapter will share ideas about determination, perseverance, dedication—all characteristics of your will—the "temperature of your desire."

TWO

Where There Is a Will

*"The greatest gift which God in His bounty bestowed
in creating, and the most conformed to His own
goodness, and that which He prizes the most,
was the freedom of the will, with which the
creatures that have intelligence
are endowed."*

—*Dante Alighieri*
(1265-1321)

YES. WHERE THERE IS A WILL THERE IS A WAY.

Those who, throughout the ages, have had the uncanny sensitivity to probe deeply into life's mysteries, have always perceived the will and the freedom of the will as the fundamental force affecting the human condition.

Your world is one of your own making, a limitless opportunity awaiting your determination to possess it, as evidenced by the stirring view from the pen of C.G. Leland; "One who can develop one's will has the power to realize very extraordinary states of mind, faculties, talents or abilities never suspected to be within reach. All that has been attributed to the invisible world without, lies, in fact, within, and the magic key is the will."

It has been written, "The achievements of history have been the choices, the determinations, the creations of the human will; no one can ever estimate the power of will. It's a part of the divine nature. The development of one's willpower is of supreme moment

9

in relation to success in life. Most people fail, not through lack of education or agreeable personal qualities, but from lack of will."

Dr. Russell Conwell, founder of Temple University, would agree. He states: "There has been altogether too much talk about the secret of success. Success has no secret. Her voice is forever ringing through the marketplace and crying in the wilderness, and the burden of her cry is one word—will."

"The Power of Will" by Frank Channing Haddock, Ph.D., published first in 1907, became a phenomenon of the publishing business. After much searching I found a copy. Mine was from a printing of 25,000 that was the 302nd edition. Imagine 302 editions when there were no talk shows, mega bookstores, author tours and all the promotion, glitz, and hype that the book Barnums use today to sell their wares. Haddock writes: "As the present edition goes to press there is an army of students of 'Power of Will.' This is a record unequaled by any other book of a similar nature in the history of literature. Thousands of warm letters of praise have been received from people in all walks of life who are being helped to a quick realization of their most cherished ambitions."

Obviously there was a growing hunger in the public's appetite for the subject matter. Could it be that the human will seemed more important then than it does now?

With no medical benefits, social security, unemployment compensation, welfare, food stamps, support groups, therapies, or the whole array of labor-saving devices, the only salvation for comforts, security, and, yes, survival, was the human will. Yet, strip away all the seductive illusions of how we can achieve mastery over one's life, and the ultimate means of personal empowerment is, still today, the "power of the will."

THE IMPACT OF WILL

The will has been defined as the "soul's sense of self-direction." The human will is the soul itself shaping one's character, integrity, and divinity. The will brings about restoration, transformation, and healing. Although the will itself does not heal, it will attract those forces or rituals that do heal.

Haddock asserts that, "all genuine cases of healing by metaphysical methods are the results of suggestion by self or others by means of a great law as yet little understood." There has never been a healing, no matter how miraculous, that does not have behind it a human will.

Years ago a man left a city to spend his last days on the desert. Diagnosed as being terminally ill, he was content to settle into a barren shack on the fringe of a settled community. Driven by an instinct unlike that of the dying, he sought hardship rather than comfort. Every day he trudged several miles up and down sandy slopes lugging his water supply.

The survival impulses were unleashed on his hut-like home. Day-long efforts were turned into cupboards, latches, innovations, and finally, added rooms.

Uninhibited by architectural restraints, this recluse lived years longer creating what was finally a gobbledygook castle of crannies, nooks, sanctuaries, and devices of his own contrivance.

Here was an extended life reborn and nourished by will. Obsessed not by death but by life, this desert hermit put new shapes and forms into being.

There can be no greatness, no meaning, no personal empowerment, no sustenance of the body or mind without human will. Hugo, the French literary giant of the 18th century, wrote, "People do not lack strength; they lack will."

Haddock writes: "Whatever you are, aside from incurable heredity, is due to your use of the will. If your character is weak or strong it is because you have permitted it to become so. All higher powers inhere in the will. They are nothing without the will. They come to perfection through the will. The will is the center from which all powers radiate to the circle of the perfected personality. The basic purpose of life is self-determined unfoldment. The control factor in such unfoldment is will.

"Your majestic endowment, your will, constitutes the high privilege granted to you to test how much you will make of yourself. It is clothed with powers which will enable you to obtain the greatest of all possessions—self-possession. If you can have this you can have any other possession you want.

"Your mind is your sole workshop for success in this world. The skill with which you transform the mind's energy into visible reality all rests with your will."

THE WILL EMPOWERS

Your will can be developed and strengthened. From that process you become personally empowered. This book is devoted to that objective.

Personal empowerment is formed from the will. A noted pioneer of the subject at the turn of the century was Richard Ingalese who wrote, "Will determines the direction and intensity of thought. Will determines the nature of thought, whether it be constructive or destructive, positive or negative, knowing the functions of this tremendous force, which in its higher aspects is latent in most persons, you can see how essential it is that it should be awakened; for, like the muscles of the body, will grows stronger with use. It is left with each of us to determine whether we shall remain infirm of purpose and weak in will, or awaken, and arouse this force and use it for our upbuilding."

THE WILL CAN BE DEVELOPED

Haddock would agree: "The spirit that summons, guides, and controls is the soul's mysterious power of self-direction—the will. And this power is susceptible of being developed. Much of life's suffering is due to the fact that the will is neither developed nor trained by conscious intelligent effort.

"The education of the will should be begun, contradictory as it may seem, by assuring yourself you can do what you wish to do. By 'what you wish to do' we mean the ambitions proper to your intelligence and place in life. Not to set yourself an impossible task, is half the battle.

"The education of the will is really of far greater importance, as shaping the destiny of the individual, than that of the intellect. It is by doing, that we learn to do; by overcoming, that we learn to overcome; by obeying reason and conscience, that we learn to obey; and every right action which we cause to spring out of pure principles, whether by authority, precept or example, will have a greater weight in the formation of character than all the theory in the world."

The venerable Harvard psychologist William James suggests that "nothing schools the will, and renders it ready for effort in this complex world, better than accustoming it to face disagreeable things. Do something occasionally for no other reason than you would rather not do it. Such effort is like the insurance you pay on your house. You have something to fall back upon in time of trouble. A will schooled in this way is always ready to respond, no matter how great the emergency."

Perhaps this is what Charles Kingsley had in mind in 1855 when he wrote in *Westward Ho:* "Thank God every morning when you get up that you have something to do that day which must be done, whether you like it or not. Being forced to work, and forced to do your best, will breed in you temperance and self-control, diligence and strength of will, cheerfulness and content, and a hundred virtues which the idle never know."

Strengthening of the will is achieved only by deliberate intent. Often that fact remains hidden. For we start out in life kicking and screaming and crying to get the things we need. Many continue kicking and screaming and crying and asking, "What is the world going to do about me?" Bedeviled by that enigma they moan, groan, manipulate, run away, criticize, complain, blame, and demand as the will becomes more and more enfeebled. Any person who is swinging at the end of a rope of addictions, turmoil and suffering is, without variance, one whose will is buried, shriveled or pushed aside. If fortunate, those who are wayworn and emptied by these realities, become blessed with one boisterous "Aha!" In that wondrous instant they become aware of what the world is going to do about them. And the answer is, "Nothing."

At that moment, hopefully, a slumbering will awakens and starts working to attract the joy, success, love, and wholeness that is inherent in life. That, also, is the beginning of self-empowerment.

SELF-CULTIVATION OF THE WILL

Training and strengthening your will is your personal responsibility. Sweep aside the victimizing beliefs of blame, self-pity, apathy, and limitation. H. Emilie Cady in her classic *Lessons In Truth* proclaims: "Wrong beliefs arise only in the human mind; we can, by persistent effort of the will, change the beliefs, and by this means alone entirely change our troublesome circumstances and bodily conditions."

Haddock suggests that the training of the will starts with: "'I resolve to will.' After a time that phrase is in the air, blows with the wind, shines in star and sun, sings with rivers and seas, whispers with dreams of sleep and trumpets through the hurly-burly of day. Eventually it becomes a feeling of achievement saturating consciousness."

In our seminars we have a similar resolve proven effective by thousands. It is the simple affirmation repeated often, "I am. I can. I will." I'll explain the further use of that and other affirmations in a later chapter. But you need not wait. You can begin now by repeating, "I am. I can. I will."

Another affirmation comes from the impassioned will of William Henley, a writer who knew what Shakespeare called a "sea of troubles." At an early age he contacted a tubercular ailment that resulted in the loss of one foot. Saving the other one meant a series of operations and endless months stretched out on a cot in the Edinburgh Infirmary. That was a way of life with Henley—disease, pain, suffering, and poverty. When his father died the young writer took on the support of his mother and five brothers and sisters. He stood by in helpless grief as his only child died after a long and baffling illness. Finally, after an accident, he too wasted away over weeks of agony and distress. But implanted within that life was an indomitable will and from that courageous heart came these words, one of the most celebrated poems of our time:

> *"Out of the night that covers me,*
> *Black as the pit from pole to pole,*
> *I thank whatever gods may be,*
> *For my unconquerable soul."*

So, at times when the world seems to be closing in around you, try bolstering your will with Henley's suggestion; "Thank God for my unconquerable soul!"

THE RIGHTEOUSNESS OF WILL

The human will becomes divinely self-empowering only when it is aligned with God's will. The human will has been unjustly criticized as being evil, opposed to God's will. That is true only when the will has been thought to be above God's will or contaminated with viciousness, hatred, sin, or arrogance. "By nothing is the will so easily disorganized as by that of evil," according to Haddock.

Life is an expression of the self-contemplation of a divine intelligence called God. God is infinitely, eternally good. Therefore, the human soul is good. It is moral. It is righteous. The human will is the soul's energy for self-direction. When set in harmony with God's will it becomes synergistic, self-empowering.

Jim Rosemergy, spiritual leader and author, asserts: "Many believe the body is the meeting place of two wills—our will and God's will. Our will is unified with God's will when we know what it means to be spiritually whole. One of the reasons sickness still dominates the human scene is that our will and God's will have not been in concert. Let us begin to open ourselves to wholeness. When we ask for an awareness of our spiritual wholeness, God's will and our will are joined."

Haddock, inspired by some ethereal sensitivity, writes: "The cultivation of the will involves the moral quality and symmetry of the soul as sustaining relations to its Deity. Righteousness alone justifies the existence of the human will. The mood of righteousness is bent on ascertaining the moral quality of actions. It is the loftiest of moods having reference to will. It clears the mind, uncovers all motives, illumines the judgment, inspires resolution, induces perseverance, arouses the understanding and guides the reason. The mood of righteousness governs the universe—that is its superiority—and exhibits the strength of an Almighty Will."

The energy of willpower has been introduced because it is the foundation upon which self-empowerment is built. Your dedication to the assignments is dependent on your will.

The eight assignments not only empower but they are exercises which train and strengthen the will. To emphasize the value of such exercises let's go back, once more, to Frank Channing Haddock: "The will grows by exercise. Each form of its activity becomes more perfect by practice. So, practice the exercises. They will gradually establish in your conscious mind the feeling that you are living and acting according to infallible law. You will soon realize that you are directing your own course—that you can deliberately proceed this way or that, as you choose. And with the unfolding of this higher consciousness there will come forward the deep inner confidence that you are your own master—that you are unswayed by external forces which drive most people with ruthless jocularity."

Ella Wheeler Wilcox said it this way:

> *One ship drives east, and another west*
> *With the self-same winds that blow;*
> *'Tis the set of the sails*
> *And not the gales,*
> *That decides the way we go.*
> *Like the winds of the sea are the ways of fate,*
> *As they voyage along through life;*
> *'Tis the will of the soul*
> *That decides its goal,*
> *And not the calm or the strife.*

∽ PERSONAL EMPOWERMENT ∾

ASSIGNMENT NUMBER ONE

"Surrender and Connect"

THREE

Getting Through to Your Divinity

YOU HAVE WITHIN YOU A GOD-CHILD AND AN EGO-CHILD. I use the term "child" because they are both children who grow with nurturing, care, understanding, and training. They will always be with you as children with you as their caretaker, responsible for their maturity.

The God-child is, in truth, the child of God and is very wise. It is well that you allow this child to be the center of your life, guiding and determining your destinies.

The God-child's heart is forever gently longing to return home. So, after walking you through the valleys, mountains, and meadows of your life, the God-child will, at some time, take you by your hand and lead you back to its home and your eternal peace. Then you "shall know as you are also known."

Next is your Ego-child.

The "ego" has for ages been an enigma to the philosophers, sages, and intellectual seers, each having a slightly different interpretation. So you will find a variance of definitions depending on whether you're talking with Saint Paul, who knew it as the "carnal mind," or Sigmund Freud with a profound psychological delineation, or a Greek mythologist telling the tale of Narcissus.

Remember the story?

Narcissus, in ancient Greek mythology, was the son of the river god Cephisus. Proud and handsome, he was the object of many girls' love. The nymph Echo was one of them. But Narcissus was indifferent towards such affection. Echo was so hurt by his coldness that all but her voice faded away.

The gods, angered at this, condemned Narcissus to fall in love with his own reflection in a pool of water. He became so much in love with himself that he could not leave the pool. There he died as he gazed unceasingly at his reflection and was changed into the flower named "Narcissus," which became a symbol of heartless beauty.

So we have the term "narcissism" defining intense self-love and self-admiration which is the prelude for being labeled as "egotistical."

Such a diversity of definitions gives me license, I believe, to render my own description of the Ego-child.

I look upon the Ego-child as the carrier of good tidings, ways of valuing one's life. Perhaps all forms of life have "egos." Why else would a weed fight for its life from a few grams of dirt in the hair-like crevice of a rock if it did not place value on its life? Why would a rabbit run from a lion if it did not have an ego? Why wouldn't it just sit and be content to be eaten if it did not value its life? Sure, such behavior can be termed "self-preservation," but why would such a motivation exist if the self has no purpose for surviving, no pride, no self-esteem, no self-actualization, no Ego-child stimulating these characteristics?

Since pre-Biblical times there has been a similarity in how the Ego-child is perceived. It has been censored as being an inherently troublesome child blamed for most of the human turmoil, self-centeredness, and arrogance. It is accused of all sorts of deviltry, the more prominent being as a staunch and strenuous adversary of one's spiritual self, the God-child. So the Ego-child is thought to be the burdensome obstacle to finding bliss, peace, and spiritual enlightenment.

I'm troubled with that. This would seem to provoke a sort of self-hate for a part of one's humanness, creating a battleground between the mortal and the spiritual—a constant squabble and bickering between the God-child and the Ego-child.

The Ego-child is very much a part of life. And who created life? Would the Mother Creator, Divine Love, who has given birth to all life, implant such a destructive device in the human soul, the beloved? I think not.

In the Mundaka Upanishad it is written: "Like two golden birds perched on the selfsame tree, ultimate friends, the ego and the self dwell in the same body. The former eats the sweet and sour fruits of the tree of life, while the latter looks on in detachment."

John White, noted author and educator, writes in New Thought: "To discover the sacredness of life in the present moment is to be released from suffering into ecstasy, quiet bliss, timeless joy. (It is also to discover—surprise!—that the ego, source of all suffering, is ultimately a gift from God, indeed, an expression of God and a form of God.)"

The Ego-child can be self-empowering, providing energy, vitality, and motivation to become what one is capable of becoming, an expression of God's contemplation. The Ego-child cybernates in your soul attempting to fulfill its purpose—to self-actualize your uniqueness, your humanness, within the circumference of your spirituality.

Unattended, the Ego-child can be exactly that—a child— immature, fearful, uncertain, needing your care, guidance, discipline, and understanding.

Romping about in the sanctuary of the mind the Ego-child is difficult to hold on to and describe—sort of like trying to explain what an onion tastes like. But there are certain characteristics that are understandable. Let's look at some of those.

THE EGO-CHILD LOOKS AT LIFE

The Ego-child views life much like a candy store or toy shop—an endless panorama of sweets and goodies and baubles and eye-sparkling delights. What is seen is wanted. Unrestrained, the wants, from childhood to old age, can increase at a reckless rate. They become the attachments and addictions that lead to futility and despair. The more the Ego-child is obsessed with wants, the more isolated it becomes from the God-child.

Those who are self-empowered have immunized themselves from the attachments of worldly treasures and surrendered to the spiritual forces within themselves. The ultimate fulfillment, the ecstasy of life, is found only by turning from wants—the delusion that having more will bring happiness—to attending to the deeper needs of life.

So the Ego-child must be taught the difference between wants and needs. Wants are frivolous, capricious desires that devour and overcome the meaningful motivation of life.

Needs, on the other hand, are soils of the soul from which more noble aspirations are grown. One does not have to abandon all, become an ascetic, or dervish, to meet needs. Simply train the Ego-child to change the urge for wants into a respect for needs.

Transform the craving for getting into the satisfaction of giving.

Transcend the want for bigger, better, and more beautiful with the less stressful need for comforts, security, and peace of mind.

Don't be hostile toward the Ego-child for its compulsion for wants. Show compassion and understanding. Teach it how to transmute the wants into needs. The Ego-child will not become weaker, but stronger, an empowering increment of wholeness. That's growth.

Like your household pet, the Ego-child has an instinctive territorial imperativeness. Your inner space is the Ego-child's territory to possess and protect. True, that might tend toward resistance to change, a closed mind, and an overzealous sense of righteousness. On the other hand, this is the armor with which one protects one's values, beliefs, integrity, and individuality. There are the charlatans, abusers, predators, cultists, cynics, campaigners, hucksters, manipulators, pessimists, and pushers—the list is endless—who would have others succumb to their pitches and pleas. So the Ego-child's territorial imperative's intent is to protect one against abuse, harassment, self-destruction, heartache, and suffering. But this hereditary instinct must be modified, tamed, and domesticated. Expand its space of concern from inner to outer. That would be sharing and loving.

The Ego-child, in its anxiousness to build self-esteem and subdue feelings of inferiority, will sometimes prod one into boasting, competing, bragging, or neglecting the significance of others—behavior that drives people away. Such inclinations are signals to step in, practice self-assurance and humility. Humility is not false modesty. It is the realization of the importance of others.

Be one in whose presence people become better. Share the energy of your Ego-child to vitalize and motivate those about you. Help others to reach out, reach up, and grow.

So, there is the God-child within you, always eager to bring truth, love, healing, peace, and compassion into your life. And then there is the Ego-child, the pillar of your humanness, but also rambunctious and aggressive which, allowed to dominate or subdue the God-child, can lead to sickness, loneliness, and despair. Therefore, the God-child and Ego-child must be reconciled, taught to go forward hand-in-hand, the God-child leading and the Ego-child following, never the other way around. For, as Goethe wrote, "Things which matter most must never be at the mercy of things which matter least."

I think of this as being a metamorphosis of atonement. Atonement is thought to be a wrenching, sacrificial event. It need not be. It can be mystical and beautiful as when Jesus proclaimed, "I am the way, the truth and the life."

When the pronoun "I" is used, it is the human, the Ego-child, speaking. Jesus did not say, "God is the way." He said "I am the way"—perfect reconciliation, atonement, an acknowledgment of the divinity of his immortality.

SURRENDER TO YOUR DIVINITY

There is a divine plan for your life. Only your God-child, often lonely and unnoticed, knows the plan and is longing to guide you along its path. So surrender. Surrender to the God-child and your spirituality.

Surrendering to the invisible, the unknown, may not be easy. The senses must be quieted from the clamor and turmoil of everyday thoughts.

Surrender may come from being exhausted by grief, pain, or despair and the utter futility of having nowhere to go but to surrender.

Surrender may mean desperately reaching out for tranquillity and peace—a soul crying out for truth rather than illusion.

Surrender may emerge from a mind weary of hypocrisy, anger, and hate.

Surrender may be a way of escaping from a world driven by greed, competition, and the raucous chatter of materialism.

Or surrender may happen by being overwhelmed by the grandeur of a mountain crest or a setting sun.

Surrender may be a flash of ecstatic awareness, a vision of clarity and eternal truth.

Surrender may mean setting aside for a moment all disturbances of the mind, a prelude to prayer perhaps—a time of meditation when the mind is opened and all resistance ceases.

SURRENDER AND LISTEN

Listen very closely; the voice of the God-child will speak softly, but will say something like this, no matter who you are or in what part of the planet you live: "I come to you from your spiritual center where there are no limitations, no bounds, no circumference to your allness and good—where all things are possible. God is not somewhere out there, but in here. I speak, not as a visitor, but the guardian of your soul."

Yes, that is the message. God is not somewhere out there but in here. There are those who have surrendered and listened and the world changed.

The most eventful periods in the history of civilization were when the human mind was illumined with the revelation that God is not out there but in here.

Out of the ancient Hindu scriptures emerged the doctrine of Brahman, the universal self and its identity with the individual soul. In the Upanishads, the wellspring of Hindu religion, we find, "He who is bewildered is bewildered because he sees not the creator abiding within himself."

Several hundred years after that message was written it was confirmed by Siddhartha Gautama, who was raised in luxury in Nepal. He renounced the world he knew to search for peace and solutions to human suffering. At the age of 35, while meditating under a pipal tree at Bodh Gaya, he achieved supreme enlightenment, an awareness of a divine presence. He became known as the Buddha. Thus was Buddhism founded, the central concept being that there is a potential Buddha-hood, purity and spirituality, innate in all beings.

Five hundred years later, into a world steeped with religious dogma and ritual, came a young lad named Jesus, a carpenter's son. At an early age he showed an interest in the religious and philosophical issues of the scriptures and prophets.

And then one day it happened, we know not when. A magnificent transformation took place in the consciousness of Jesus— from the mortal to the spiritual. From some eternal presence within came the revelation of his divinity. Empowered by this great discovery, Jesus began performing works which were viewed as miracles. Since it was believed by most that humanity was separate from God, many saw Jesus as having unusual omnipotent powers far beyond the reach of themselves. That, however, was not his message. His profound awareness perceived all of humankind to be divine, endowed with a spiritual unity with God.

"He that believeth in me, the works that I do shall he do also; and greater works than these shall he do."

Some 600 years after the birth of Christianity, one of the great prophets of history, Muhammed, sensed a spiritual awakening when he reached the age of forty. Stirring within were revelations from God that would be the visions of a new religion. These were set forth in the Koran and became the basis of Islam, which, for millions of Muslims, meant the submission to, or having peace with, God.

Examine the words and teachings of these spiritually enlightened and they are not unlike those of the mystics and sages of all ages. The message is awesomely simple. God is not out there but in here. There is no separation.

YOUR SPIRITUAL CENTER

Within you is a spiritual center, the source of your divinity, healing, wholeness, and eternal life. It is recognized in nearly all of the great religions as the liberating force from suffering and bondage. In Hinduism, for example, it is known as the Brahman, in Christianity as the Christ, and Buddhism as Nirvana.

To me it is a God-child; it touches my soul, it speaks, it embraces me, heals me, carries my burdens, and softens my pains. It is more than a nebulous spirit without form or feeling.

Yes, I can talk to it and it speaks. I once requested, "Take me to God." And the God-child answered, "I have. Didn't you know?"

That meant I hadn't learned to listen. Be still and listen. Don't expect a thunderous voice from the clouds, words etched in stone, an angel floating down from the heavens or a lightning-like burst of enlightenment. The God-child's presence may be so tender and gentle you may not even be aware of its soft breeze that is filling the sails of your soul. You may feel you have a guardian angel watching over you, and, upon occasion you say, "I don't know what made me do that."

Yes. Learn to listen. For the God-child, so dear and so merciful and so calm, speaks softly, very softly. You may hear just a murmur, a whisper in the inner ear for only a moment, at times, and then the voice disappears. Or you may feel an intuitive nudge, a notion that prompts you to think, "something told me to do that." Or perhaps you have an instinctive urge, a compulsion to act in a way that defies reason or logic. You might have a vision, a darting picture in the mind's eye, even a dream, perchance, followed by words tumbling through a mind numbed by sleep. Let me share an example.

It was on a trip, a casual one, typical of many. I flew into Seattle, arriving in early evening after a three-hour flight. I checked into the hotel, read the local newspaper, and went to the restaurant for a late dinner.

When I returned to the room I crawled into bed, put a pillow behind my back and started making notes about the next day's business meeting. But I was weary—brain weary. So I put the pad and pen aside and read a bit out of the Gideon Bible. Not for long. I dozed off, slipping into a deep sleep.

Sometime in the center of night I dreamt. It was a lovely dream with a panoramic vision of flowers and trees, and mountain slopes. From somewhere came a voice. Then I woke blurred by sleep. The scene disappeared. But the voice continued. I wrote down the words.

"Our Power which is in all,
Perfect is your being.
Your love has come,
Your will be done,
In body as it is in spirit.
Provide us this day with our daily needs,
And forgive us our intolerances
As we forgive those who are intolerant towards us;
And lead us not into false beliefs,
But deliver us from fear, doubt, and hate.

> *For yours is the One Mind, the One Power,*
> *the One Spirit forever."*

Rarely do we realize the significance of events when they happen. Time reveals that. I was not fully aware of the depth to which the words I wrote down would touch my life. As time went by I repeated them frequently. They always brought comfort and peace. At one time, which I will share later, I hung on to them frequently as anchors for my wholeness.

Ah! The God-child is indeed very wise. You will cherish this wisdom as you dance with the mysticism of life. You will most certainly learn new steps.

CONNECT WITH THE POWER

Yes! Surrender and listen. Then connect. Connect with your spiritual center. That is somewhat like plugging an electric cord into an outlet, the power source. By connecting, plugging in to your spiritual center, you become empowered.

It is only through connecting that you become aware of your true identity. You can't learn it from a book, a sermon, a seminar, or a single event. You must resurrect your own salvation by seeking and searching and reaching down into your mind, and letting your God-child lead you to your spiritual center. Then you will find your divinity, the infinite nature of your soul; each time you connect is a step forward in your spiritual quest; you will never go back to where you were.

To connect you are given few directions but many choices. Let me suggest one that may be helpful. This came to me by being with Norman Vincent Peale, a wonderfully kind and humble man. To be in his presence was to absorb his positive energy. He didn't always possess that. He told this story years ago.

"When I was a teenager, I was introverted, shy, and didn't think much of myself," he said. "One day I was complaining about my problems to my mother. She listened patiently and then told me, 'Norman, you're made in the image of God.' And that's all she said.

"That struck home with me. I'm made in the image of God. That's really something. I'm made in the image of God. God doesn't feel inferior. God isn't shy or bashful. I don't have to be."

That was a turning point in his life. He devoted his ministry to the "…power of positive thinking."

You are made in the image of God. I paraphrased that into an affirmation that I have said hundreds of times.

"I'm a reflection of God's perfection."

Say it. "I'm a reflection of God's perfection." It has rhythm and rhyme. Say it again…and again…and again… Say it when you're walking. Say it when you're waiting in line or at a stop sign. Say it in the morning, say it during the day. Say it when you're sleepless in the darkness of night with your troubled mind.

Say it when your self-esteem has bottomed out, or when you're struggling with your addictions, feel guilty, are overweight, sick, kicked out of a job, dumped from a relationship, or mired in a swamp of despair. Repeat it over and over. "I'm a reflection of God's perfection." God won't be offended. Really!

You have nothing at risk. Saying those words won't make you hurt more than you're hurting. Repeat the phrase enough times and you're going to penetrate that gray cloud of insane clutter that you've allowed to gather and obscure your spiritual center. Repeat the affirmation enough times and a lacy aura begins forming in your consciousness to a presence that truly is a "reflection of God's perfection"—a spiritual being created in the image of God.

The Purpose of Prayer

Repeating those words may be a way of preparing your mind for the deeper rituals of connecting known as prayer. What is prayer? Why do you pray? Do you ask God to repair your life or to repair you?

Are prayers exercises of pleading, begging, and petitioning God for favors and benevolent gifts? Is prayer a last resort where all other efforts have failed? Is prayer a strategy for convincing, persuading, or manipulating God into fixing something or someone that you believe needs fixing? Can God really be influenced by such human intervention?

God never stops being God, does not need awakening, informing, or changing. God is perfect. Human prayers cannot alter that perfection.

God does not give. God is.

Do you, for example, pray to be loved? You are. God is love. You are surrounded and immersed in love. There can be no greater love than already exists. Do you pray for God to give more than is already given? Pleading for love is like sitting in the darkness and begging for the warmth of sun beams. The sun can give no more than it is giving; it shows no preference and plays no favorites. But you must get out of the darkness into the sunlight. Do it with God's love. Prayer is a way of connecting—getting into the sunlight of God's love.

Do you pray to be healed? God has already done that. Healing is not a process; it is a revelation. There are not many ways to heal. Like the law of gravity there is only one force, one law of healing. The objectives of all medical technology and doctor's skills are to connect with that law.

Surrender and connect to your spiritual center and it's perfection. Physical and mental restoration will follow.

Do you pray for abundance and prosperity? God has provided for that. The universe is an unlimited source of good. Belief in limitation, scarcity and lack are frauds of human thought, indications, perhaps, of a poverty of the spirit.

Connect with your spiritual center. Nourish the spiritual self; set it free to flourish, serve, and share. Become aware of its boundless nature; abundance will follow.

Do you pray for loved ones? They are already in God's care. They, too, must be connected to the spiritual forces within them. Your prayers can help by clearing the obstructions, seeing their minds as surrendering and connecting. There is only one mind, one cosmic intelligence that is infinitely all. Your mind is an individual expression of this one sea of consciousness. Your prayers can have a transcendent effect on the spiritual strength of another. Envision and proclaim the spiritual perfection of others.

Do you pray for God to remedy the chaos, futility, and ruptured dreams of your outer world? God has done that. Divine order is a virtual fountainhead of joy, harmony and contentment. Your spiritual center has been endowed with this atmosphere. You are a reflection of God's perfection.

It is futile to spend time praying and pleading to God for works that have already been done. You don't have to tell God how to be God; nor can you change God by your petitions. God knows your needs, has always known them, far better than you do.

Now I understand the response I received when I said to my God-child, "Take me to God." And the reply was, "I already have. Didn't you know?"

THE POWER OF PRAYER

It is useless to plead vigorously for God to change what is causing our miseries while we hang tenaciously on to the real causes within us.

Prayer is not a way of changing what is outside ourselves but, rather, to change what is inside ourselves. Prayer purifies the mind, clears and opens it to the omnipotent allness of God. It is to go to the deepest level of consciousness and be enlightened, to find truth, reality and become fully alive. Connect. Experience the reverie of prayer.

Cleanse your mind of un-God-like thoughts. Just as oil and water do not mix, so a mind clinging to anger, hatred, anxiety, cynicism, doubt, or greed will find difficulty in connecting.

Before praying, quiet your mind, let it be calm. Be still and let the peace of God's love saturate your consciousness. Yield. Let your thoughts rise above the events of the day into a sea of tranquillity, a place where there is no separation from God. Just as a plant turns to the sun and absorbs its energy, so your words will draw the Infinite Power into your consciousness. Whatever you declare or affirm in this atmosphere of thought will be manifested.

PRACTICE POSITIVE PRAYER

Prayers that get results are positive affirmations of spiritual truths. They are not filled with "give me," "help me," "heal me," or pleas and petitions. Rather, they are declarations of "I am." As the prophet Joel long ago declared, "Let the weak say, I am strong."

All that you need, your unlimited good, you already have in your spiritual center. Claim it and accept it by your prayerful words. Surrender and connect. Sprinkle your prayers with affirmations like the following—some you may want to repeat many times. Know that you don't have to believe them to say them; God understands that. Conviction and belief often follow with repetition and demonstration.

AFFIRMATIVE PRAYER

I celebrate the presence of God in all, through all, as all.

I am restored by the healing presence of God flowing in and through my body.

I surrender to the in-dwelling spirit and allow it to work through me for my greatest good.

I rest in God's love, free from worry, anxiety, and fear.

There is one Power, one Spirit, one Mind, and that Mind is my mind now.

I am one with the Divine Order of the universe and power that draws the planets through space with effortless ease.

God's love nurtures, protects, and empowers me.

I go forth this day striving to fulfill my highest purpose to honor God's presence.

Every cell of my body is created, sustained, and restored as the perfect idea of God—complete, whole, and indestructible.

I harmonize all my relationships with God's love.

I experience abundance, prosperity, and joy by my awareness of God's infinite good.

I dwell in the secret place of the most high, my spiritual center, a refuge from sickness and suffering.

I surrender to the allness and perfection of God.

Divine love floods my consciousness, dissolving all that is unlike God.

In this stillness I am aware of my oneness with all life.

The spiritual currents that guide and direct all cosmic substance are now flowing through me. I yield to the vastness of this force.

I surrender and connect to the light and love of God.

I find peace and comfort in the majesty of these moments with God.

I strive to fulfill the image of my spiritual self held in Infinite Mind.

The healing power of God moves in and through me, restoring my wholeness.

Centered in God, my life unfolds with Divine Order.

Adversity is a gift that will reveal my opportunity for spiritual growth and learning.

God lives, moves, and is ever-present as my spiritual center.

I go now to my spiritual center where the solution I seek is seeking me.

THE FIRST ASSIGNMENT

The first assignment for self-empowerment is "Surrender and Connect."

You are not a helpless mortal encased in a body of flesh and bones seeking to become spiritual. You have never been other than an unlimited image of a perfect spiritual idea. There is within you a spiritual center, a divine presence, which is the core of your being. "Be ye, therefore, perfect." Know this and you become empowered.

This is reality, truth, and freedom from bondage. Anything that stands against this, whether it be sickness, suffering, despair, or pain is powerless, false, and transient.   You don't see yourself like that? Do you live with your anger, your hopelessness, and your pain, in an unloving world of violence, hate, and indifference? Let's think about that.

Your anger is not you.

Your guilt is not you.

Your weaknesses are not you.

Your doubts and fears are not you.

Your sickness and pain are not you.

Your irritation, frustrations, and aggravations are not you.

Your self-condemnation is not you.

Your possessions are not you.

Those are illusions masquerading as reality. They are phantoms created and defended by the surface texture of the mind. In truth, however, you are a spiritual being, free of all imperfections, templed in a human body. Connecting with that presence can be the dearest and noblest of life's experiences, a way of casting out the ghosts that haunt the mind.

Realize that surrendering and connecting is a lifetime, never-ending adventure climbing stairs that start in darkness and emerge into the light that radiates life. Know that with each step comes a greater peace, comfort, and personal empowerment.

But know, too, that if the hunger and need are there and you seek, you will be shown. Your Creator did not lock the divine presence within you never to be discovered. You will be led.

"You will seek me and find me; when you seek me with all your heart, I will be found by you." (Jeremiah 29:13-14)

The lesson is clear. Surrender and connect to your spiritual center. That is the source of your divinity, healing, higher power, wholeness and eternal life—and, most certainly, personal empowerment.

You will become a healer—not only for yourself but others; you will help to heal the planet, restoring it to purity and goodness.

Your effort, so seemingly small, will be preserved in perpetuity. You don't believe that? "Not me," you say, "A grain of sand on an endless beach." But that does not diminish your significance.

Why not let God decide how that which flows from your spiritual center fits into the oneness of all life? Just work on this first assignment: "Surrender and Connect." And trust, as these words by an unknown writer suggest: "When the charge or care of anything rests upon you, God ceases to be a God of peace. Bear not a single care, one is too much for you; the work is mine, and mine alone and yours is—trust in Me."

∽ PERSONAL EMPOWERMENT ∽

ASSIGNMENT NUMBER TWO

"Be Miracle-Minded"

FOUR

The Magic of Miracles

LET'S THINK OF A MIRACLE AS BEING ANY EVENT BEYOND HUMAN UNDERSTANDING OR EXPLANATION.

You are a miracle.

You began as a single egg, one among incalculable numbers, all competing for fertilization, with only one succeeding. With odds beyond definition, yours was the single triumph, the end chain of synchronistic events going back millions of years.

The miracles continue. You breathe. You hear. You see. You eat; your food goes through a process that would take laboratories days to simulate. Millions of body cells, each a miracle in itself, are constantly being created all with appointed missions of maintaining your life.

You are, essentially, a universe within a universe. You exist on a whirling planet working harmoniously with a distant sun—dynamic energies calibrated by omnipotent intelligence down to the minute and meter to sustain the life force that is you.

Every moment of every day you are immersed in and surrounded by miracles. Untold miracles, beyond human anticipation or comprehension, are waiting to unfold in your life. If you wait for them to be explained by science or logic they will sink into oblivion. Why not accept them?

Why not allow miracles to flourish in your life? Why not be "miracle-minded"? That, then, is the second assignment for self-empowerment. "Be miracle-minded."

To be miracle-minded is to set aside skepticism, doubt, and pessimism. Open your mind. You don't have to understand or depend on miracles. But don't resist them. Accept them. You will find them happening with greater frequency as you work on your first assignment: "surrender and connect."

Shift your perception to miracle mindfulness. Clear your mind. Open it to the wonders of life—the mystery, mysticism, romance, the divine life force throbbing through the universe as a supporting mechanism to make all things possible for you. That's the magic of miracles. Don't miss out. Be miracle-minded.

Expect a miracle! "But that's not reality," you say. What is reality? Reality is your perception of the world. There's also a little filtering process in your brain cells termed "selective perception." Your mind sees only what it chooses to see. Why not choose to see miracles? Why not make them your reality? Life is a wonder. That's reality. Why not perceive it with child-like reverie, seeking and finding miracles? Each day, then, becomes more fun and exciting—and, yes, miraculous.

ONLY WEEKS TO LIVE

Miracles are often associated with healings. Recently my staid and conservative doctor looked over my charts and said, "Bob, you are a miracle."

I did not disagree. For I have tried to be miracle-minded. The lessons I have learned that prompted his remark started several years before.

My upbeat life was curdling. Setbacks. Soured relationships.

Ideas that flopped. Nothing seemed to be going right. Life was losing some of its sparkle. My attitude was OK, positive, but my body was soggy—lethargic, weary, not always functioning as it should.

A vacation in Hawaii would fix everything, I thought. Clear the mind. Get the body in shape. So I was off to Hawaii. But there I grew worse, steadily. I went to see a friend, Dr. Renn, a well-known physician in the islands.

He did the usual examination and tests, which he sent to the laboratory. The lab sent them back by messenger marked "crisis." The doctor called me to his office.

Gently he spoke. "I have gone over all the test results very carefully. Frankly, I don't know how you had the strength to come in here. You want me to be honest with you. So I must tell you. I believe you have only a few weeks to live, six at the most."

We talked. Much more diagnostic work was essential, requiring immediate hospitalization. But I wanted desperately to get back home. In fact, insisted on it. So, packed in a wheelchair, I was hustled onto the next flight out.

Arriving in Minneapolis, I went directly into intensive care in the hospital.

LESSONS FROM ADVERSITY

The next three years were spent in and out of hospitals—a dozen operations, some minor, some major—dialysis-therapies—X-rays—biopsies—CAT scans—ultrasounds—and, finally, a kidney transplant.

What was wrong? Some things could be explained, some could not. But this is not a documentary to describe an inch-thick medical history. That's not where I am. As doctors would use their medical terms, I would promptly dismiss them from my mind.

Those are labels, words, with symptoms of destructive characteristics. To accept them mentally is to give them power. To believe them is to experience them. There is a diabolical invitation to the old prophecy: "That which I greatly fear has come upon me."

Struggling with medical prognoses, terms, and mind-sets for sicknesses was one of my lessons in itself. A friend, Frank, recently said to me, "I thought for a while we were going to lose you. But you're a fighter. You fought for your life and won."

No, Frank. I learned not to fight. Yes, during my lifetime I fought a lot of skirmishes in a career of management, people, problems, and ambitions. I'm a slow learner, Frank. Maybe it took a dozen operations to teach me how to be non-resistant.

All I would be doing is putting my mind in a turmoil trying to fight illness. I would be a David battling a giant I couldn't even see.

Using my mind to fight illness would be futile. I became aware that healing is done through the mind, not by it. That's very important. You don't know how to heal your body. Healing is done through the mind, not by it.

You don't accept that? Then explain how a lowly scab is formed to protect a wound. Or how is a broken bone mended? The mind you think with can create illness, but, at best, it is only a co-facilitator for healing. Once that is accepted you can practice non-resistance. That was a valuable lesson for me. Because being non-resistant not only supports the restoration process in the body but is also a wondrous strategy for daily affairs. We have so much "fight" in our language; "fighting traffic," "fighting a cold," "fighting for what is right," "fight back."

Do you find a tendency to put on your mental battle garb every day to go out and joust in the contests of life? Is it really a "rat race" out there, as some say, plagued with forays in a cold, competitive world? Must we fight our way through sickness, distress, and adversity? Only if that is perceived as reality.

Non-resistance. Yielding. Being flexible. Practicing humility. Isn't that what we have been considering? Surrender and connect. Fighting is totally different from "not accepting." I realized I did not have to accept an ominous condition because I was not fighting it. I simply did not accept all of the dire predictions and medical terms I heard. I didn't fight. I didn't argue. I didn't let fear cannibalize every thought. I became non-resistant.

Each adversity became an opportunity. Some of the deeper meanings of life began to surface. Truths emerged. There is no condition that cannot be healed. All things really are possible.

I became miracle-minded. I expected miracles.

PRACTICING EMPOWERMENT STRATEGIES

I used what lessons of personal empowerment I had learned. I held mental pictures in my mind. I pictured myself walking the beach at Maui with the sun creeping over the crest of Haleakala. And dancing with Nadine. Cruising the seas. Playing golf. I saw myself on the first tee at Hazeltine National Golf Club striking the ball pure and solid down the middle of the fairway. I played some spectacular rounds in my imagination, never once hooking or slicing or missing a putt! My mental pictures were clear and vivid, recalling favorite incidents with favorite friends. I never thought about how or when, only that I was fully restored and alive.

Visualizing is a way of seeing ourselves as reflecting the images of perfection held in our spiritual centers. Remember? "I'm a reflection of God's perfection." We'll study the techniques of visualizing in a later chapter. It is deeply self-empowering.

Affirmations were my constant companions. I repeated some many times, not parrot-like, but with care and respect for the value of each word.

I spent weeks at home sitting upright, pain preventing me from lying down. In the hospital, I was often restricted in any movement by surgical wounds and medical devices attached to the body.

Of special significance was the gift that I had received in Seattle. The prayer. Remember?

> *"Our Power which is in all,*
> *Perfect is your being.*
> *Your love has come,*
> *Your will be done,*
> *In body as it is in spirit.*
> *Provide us this day with our daily needs,*
> *And forgive us our intolerances.*
> *As we forgive those who are intolerant towards us;*
> *And lead us not into false beliefs,*
> *But deliver us from fear, doubt, and hate.*
> *For yours is the One Mind, the One Power,*
> *The One Spirit forever."*

In the loneliness of night while the world slept I pondered each phrase looking behind it for its richness and depth of meaning.

"Our Power which is in all." Our Power—the source of life, wholeness, restoration—boundless strength and goodness within us, resting, waiting for our awareness and connection.

In all—inner, outer, all there is in all that is—the trees, flowers, birds, air, sky, mountains, seas—all of life—all of the universe—wherever we are, now and forever present in each and every breath we take.

"Perfect is your being." Absolute perfection beyond human comprehension—existing, present, and being—constantly nourishing, creating, generating, preserving, and imagining perfection—the ecstasy of mind, spirit, body.

"Your love has come." Your love has saturated my consciousness—I rest in it, find comfort and tranquillity as its soothing energy quiets my fears and anguish.

"Your will be done." Your will, not my will be done…no more struggles, confusion, and physical distress from my distorted, anxiety-ridden thoughts—but your will—a will of peacefulness, unlimited good, well-being, and harmony—I surrender to it—and recognize that the meaning of life is to express your all-knowing, all-loving will, reconciling and strengthening my will.

"In body as it is in spirit." The body will reflect that which is spirit—perfection, wholeness, wellness—holding dearly to this truth will dissolve my doubt and disbelief—healing and restoration will follow—gone will be the fear, disease, and ills of the body.

"Provide us this day with our daily needs." May our needs—healing, peace, abundance, wellness, nourishment—be met today—not tomorrow or sometime but today, now.

"And forgive us our intolerances." Forgive us—the asking is the confession—the admitting to intolerances reveals the need for forgiving—removing the defenses and resistance that holds us back from loving.

"As we forgive those who are intolerant towards us." If we forgive others we will then be forgiven. What more could we ask?

"And lead us not into false beliefs." Save us from our illusions, fears, superstitions, and thoughts that separate us from love, wholeness, and perfection.

"But deliver us from fear, doubt, and hate." Cleanse our

minds of all negative thoughts—fear, doubt, and hate—the demons that disrupt, distort, or obstruct our being fully alive in the Light that knows no darkness.

"For yours is the One Mind, the One Power, the One Spirit forever." I had no alternative except to surrender, giving up worldly concerns. With surrendering and connecting came a calmness where there was no sickness, distress, or fear—only tranquillity and peace. But that is simply sensing the Divine Presence, isn't it? It's the mysticism of miracles, the significance of being miracle-minded.

THOUGHTS ABOUT HEALING

Today I am restored, healed. I am doing all the things I visualized, including golf, although, admittedly, I am not playing as well as I did in my imagination.

What creates healing and restoration? Prayer? Medical technology? Love? A higher power? Affirmations? Imaging? Or any of the therapies, disciplines, rituals, or practices existing in all cultures? We don't know, do we? We do know that there is only one law of healing. Whatever and whenever connection is made to that energy, that power, then healing will follow.

I am certain that a strong compelling force in my restoration was my constant expectation of miracles—every moment, every day. I expected a wholeness beyond human understanding and exploration. That energy, I believe, attracts the mechanisms of restoration. That is not only true of physical condition but in all of one's affairs and relationships.

Why are some healed and others not? Science has struggled with that for many years. Some information is beginning to emerge. But there is no consensus of answers. A healer was once asked why she could heal some and not others. She replied, "Some people need their illnesses."

That brought to mind a lady named Pauline, attractive, fortyish, employed in a bookstore, who came bouncing into my classroom one evening. "Hi! Remember me?" she asked. "The last time you saw me I attended your program in a wheelchair."

I asked her to stay and visit with me after class. She did. I was reminded that Pauline had spent two years in bed and five years in a wheelchair. The best hope for Pauline at one time was life in a wheelchair if she were to survive at all.

But Pauline had courage and a will. She endured her challenges, survived to walk and enjoy good health, and became an amazingly hardy person mentally.

I had my tape recorder and turned it on. So I will share Pauline's story, word for word, exactly as she told it to me.

She explained, "I suddenly realized that I was sick because I really wanted to be sick. It was something I had learned early in life. I remember as a child the only time my mother treated me gently was when I was sick. I was a whiny, fussy, unhappy child, and this was because I thought that the type of attention I got as a result was the only kind of attention in the world to get. It took years before I realized that you can decide what kind of attention you will get from other people.

"In my early twenties, I went into the hospital for the first major operation in a series of nine. And then nine years ago I became sick, seriously sick, with multiple sclerosis. I was in bed for two years and then in a wheelchair for five years. And then I realized that I rather enjoyed being in the wheelchair. Such an enormous amount of attention I got! Why, I have been in the arms of more nice men in the time of my illness than most women are in their whole life! Men would pick me up to carry me onto buses or on planes or going to sukiyaki dinners or things at church or up and down stairs. You see, this was rather nice. It was attention and it was legitimate attention, and I enjoyed that extra attention!

"And I joined a club of people who were all visibly and physically handicapped. I fitted in like a charm. I became an officer in the organization and was on a pedestal in that position. I loved that. I sometimes thought that if I had been able to get to my feet, they might not allow me to continue in that position.

"But then slowly, slowly I began to realize that I was sitting at the bottom of the stairs of life. That up at the top of the stairs was a closed door and behind that door was a whole new life. As long as I was in a wheelchair I would never be able to find out what was at the top of those stairs, behind that door. The only way to reach that door was to walk, even if I had to crawl (and that I did a few times!). As long as I got out of the wheelchair and went, I would eventually get to that door, open it, and find something better.

"So I would try struggling to my feet and moving about with the help of crutches. It took a long time after that, and I went back into the wheelchair several times; I slumped back and forth until I finally could admit to myself that the real reason I was going back to the wheelchair was to get the attention I missed!

"Once I really realized this, I was able to put away the chair and then I stopped using the crutches. Then I stayed quite a while on a cane. It was another severe tug to try being without one. The first time I went without any support was the result of having gone to a party at Easter time, and lost my cane. The next day I had to go to a part-time job at the hospital. Either I had to go without a cane or not go at all. I was trembling with fear that somebody would knock me down or I would fall down or somebody would move fast and not see me.

"And then suddenly I said to myself, 'The sun is shining and you are on a corner waiting for a bus. Is that what you want to do? Is that what you really want to do?' And I said, 'Yes, I really do!' And so I said, 'Then, forget your fear! If this is what you really want to do, do it! Forge ahead! Do the whole thing and each time it will be easier!'"

And so, ultimately, this courageous person gained a victory over her crippling oppression, a victory that started when she realized she was attracting her misfortune because she secretly wanted it. As the healer said, "Some people need their illnesses."

Looking at Lessons

Is there a lesson for you in Pauline's story? There was for me. But we all have different lessons and different teachers, don't we? Only our assignments are similar. We are given few directions but many choices. We are measured by the lessons that concern us. How well we do on our tests is determined by how well we choose our lessons.

During my periods of illness, bedridden, I did a lot of thinking, deeply and searchingly, about lessons and teachers like Pauline.

Adversity becomes so much a part of our lives that we buy into it, whether it be mental or physical. It becomes "my arthritis, my divorce, my loss, my grief, my depression, my job problem." We learn to live with our pain until we believe we can't live without it. That becomes a belief, a belief that we vigorously defend. We will even die for our beliefs as millions have demonstrated throughout time. So we die, not from the illness, but from our belief in the illness—the refusal of the human mind to let it go.

There is a certain martyrdom in suffering, a role, we feel, deserving of medals and acclaim. That can lead to pity parties to which we invite others but which no one wants to attend. Granted, there is a therapy in talking about our distress and anguish. But there comes a time to let it go, disclaim it, replace it with empowering strategies.

Yes, there was a lesson for me in Pauline's story.

As the healer said, "Some people need their illnesses." And problems. And failures. And eroded relationships. And chaos.

Invite miracles into your life. Become aware of miracle-minded people, both the famed or unknown. Their enthusiasm is inspiring and contagious. To reinforce your mission, look for stories about miracles. Like this one.

In 1622, the Spanish galleon Atocha was making her maiden voyage from Havana to Spain when she was struck by a hurricane. Swept over a barrier reef 40 miles west of Florida, the Atocha sank with a cargo of gold and silver.

Blindly optimistic, 347 years later, Mel Fisher, a retired chicken farmer from Redondo, California, went looking for the Atocha. Decades of currents, tides and shifting silt would have scattered and buried the treasure beneath miles of open sea.

Undaunted by the enormous odds against him, Fisher wrung out 16 years of tedious searching for his pot of gold. Even the loss of a son and daughter-in-law by drowning did not stop him.

Mel Fisher demonstrated how to handle losing and adversity. Put it behind you! Today is a new day! Every morning he greeted his employees with the statement, "Today's the day!"

On Saturday, July 20, 1985, he was right. Beneath five feet of silt, the watery grave of silver bars worth up to 400 million dollars was discovered!

My lesson? Start each day by saying, "This is the day! I expect a miracle today!" That doesn't mean it has to be a big one like the sun rising in the west instead of the east. Just some little ones will be fine. Look for them. For miracles are not events waiting to happen. They are what is happening around us with percussive constancy. They are simply revelations of perception, perhaps just being conscious and grateful for the miracle of life itself.

Expect a miracle. You might resist working on this assignment saying, as many others have, "Why build up false hopes? I would just be setting myself up for a letdown. Miracles seldom happen." Agreed. They don't if we don't look for them. However, expecting a miracle is never futile. Just the process is beneficial. Consider the fable told that hundreds of years ago a king had sentenced one of his slaves to death for committing a minor crime.

The slave begged, "O Master, I have a bargain to offer thee! Give me one year and I shall teach your favorite horse to fly! If I fail, then I die!"

The king pondered for a moment and then decided, "Foolish slave! What have I to lose?"

In boisterous mirth, he said, "We shall meet in the court one year from today to see the horse fly or you die!"

Afterward one of the other slaves asked the condemned man, "You fool! Why did you make a foolish bargain like that? You know you cannot make a horse fly!"

The slave answered, "Reason it this way. In one year the king might die, he might forget our bargain, he might have mercy and free me. Or if these do not happen, the horse might learn to fly!"

So, at the very least, the slave added a year to his life just by expecting a miracle!

Life is a school. This is a course in personal empowerment. There are teachers, lessons, tests—and assignments. The second assignment is: "Be miracle-minded."

Journey Begins

IT WAS A DAY TO LULL THE SENSES AND CALM THE HURRIED IMPULSES, WARM AND SUNNY—THE SPRING OF THE YEAR.

As I drove along a tree-shaded lane, words started pushing themselves through my mind, begging to be expressed.

I stopped the car and wrote them down.

I AM YOUR MASTER!
I can make you rise or fall. I can work for you or against you.
I can make you a success or failure.
I control the way you feel and the way you act.
I can make you laugh…work…love. I can make your heart sing with
joy…excitement…elation…
Or I can make you wretched…dejected…morbid…
I can make you sick…listless…
I can be as a shackle…heavy…attached…burdensome…
Or I can be as the prism's hue…
dancing…bright…fleeting…lost forever unless captured
by pen or purpose.
I can be nurtured and grown to be great and beautiful…
seen by the eyes of others through action in you.
I can never be removed…only replaced.
I am a THOUGHT.
Why not know me better?

Words flowing, uninvited, like strangers being met for the first time in the mind. What is their source? Their energy? Where do they come from? A universal mind? Cosmic consciousness? A spirit from another time residing within? A moment's habitation by an angel? An inner reservoir hidden from the consciousness? Or the God-child?

Unanswerable questions. But such illuminating experiences always have meaning and purpose. We become empowered—sometimes redirected, enlightened, or simply entrusted with an embryo whose visibility is yet unseen.

What was the intent of the words I wrote down that day? Little did I realize how they would affect my life and the lives of millions of others.

What had been revealed was the substance of life itself. For life can only be experienced by what occurs in the mind. Nothing new. For ages, it has been said many ways.

"To think is to live." (Cicero)

"Your life is what your thoughts make it." (Buddha)

How can thoughts be defined? Managed? That leads us to our attitudes. Attitudes are the ways that we think. Our attitudes towards others are the ways we think about others. Our attitudes towards our jobs are the ways we think about our jobs. Our attitudes towards ourselves are the ways we think about ourselves.

William James, the venerable Harvard psychologist, said that the greatest discovery of his generation was that "you can change your life by changing your attitudes of mind."

I was on a course of self-discovery from the day I wrote down those mystical words…"I Am Your Master."

"How can I make attitudes work for me rather than against me?" I asked myself.

THE DYNAMICS OF ATTITUDES

Relationships with others revolve about attitudes. In marriage, love brings couples together, but the success or failure of the marriage is determined by attitudes.

Our self-esteem, our highs and lows, the manner in which we accept or reject ourselves is dependent on our attitudes towards ourselves.

Attitudes calibrate one's progress in a career. Of particular interest to me at the time was a study that indicated that over 90% of a salesperson's success is dependent on mental attitudes.

I researched seminars, courses, training procedures, and other avenues of personal development. I talked with those who had attended my classes in interpersonal relationships, personality, and leadership.

The conclusions were undeniable. Although knowledge, techniques, and skills were taught, the primary benefit that participants received was the influence on their attitudes.

So I asked myself, "Why not create a course that teaches intentionally what the others do incidentally?"

That was the beginning of "Adventures In Attitudes."

HOW ADVENTURES IN ATTITUDES BEGAN

The program was first conducted in 1957 as an evening program for adults in Room 402 of the Minneapolis Vocational School. I look back with a certain reverence to that room; even with the most elastic imagination I could not possibly have predicted the phenomenon that would sprout from that unpretentious location.

I searched for material for my first program. I could find very little concerning attitude development except that similar to the Boy Scout Creed and stories like the little train that said, "I think I can; I think I can."

There were books, of course, like the "Power of Positive Thinking." But, somehow, they didn't seem to fit what I had in mind. Indeed, I didn't quite know what I had in mind. I was not clever or smart enough to lecture to others about the mystery of mysteries—human thought.

But I was led. When asked, I have often said that, although I wrote the material for the program, I most assuredly was not the author.

Starting only with my inspired verse, "I Am Your Master," the agenda had to be built from there, invented as we went along in the classroom. I did not view myself as a teacher, but, rather, as a tour guide as the participants explored the pathways of their minds. It was exactly what the name implied—an Adventure In Attitudes.

Gradually I put together projects, usually from actual experiences, that were everyday problems in life. The participants divided into small groups, discussed these and expressed their reactions and feelings. There was a magic that unfolded, strange to most, as they opened themselves to new insights from an assortment of perspectives and opinions.

The school was in the heart of the city surrounded by old rooming houses, rundown dwellings, and sparse living quarters. People came from those places because they had an unspoken need—loneliness, distress, or simply a brief respite from the hardness of their lives.

They cautiously experienced the joy of disclosure, opening up and learning from each other.

They were not put at risk; their shallow self-esteems were never threatened. There were no grades, tests, judgment, or degree of involvement required. They were people like Mrs. Kelly. She sat, secluded, in the rear of the room, too shy to even volunteer her name. She came to me after the first evening and said she didn't think she really belonged there and did not intend to come back.

I listened. We talked. I promised that if she came back she could continue sitting in the back of the room, never required to be involved, and could be a spectator rather than a participant.

She did come back and found herself slowly being embraced by the compassion of others. On the final evening Mrs. Kelly stood and thanked all her new companions for their help, encouragement, and understanding. Two weeks later, when I walked into the classroom to start my next group, who should I see in the front row? Mrs. Kelly. Bless her!

I have repeatedly found that there is a little bit of Mrs. Kelly in all of us, even the most self-reliant. Thousands of people later, the training director of one of the nation's largest corporations came to me after a few hours of the "adventure" and confessed, "I will be honest with you. I came to this program to just listen and observe, to audit it. But I found that these people were talking about me, the inner me. I was drawn in and became a part of it."

People like Mrs. Kelly went back to their homes, places of employment, churches, and friends and talked about the course. Attendance grew. Because of the increased interest of people to enroll it finally became necessary to go on a waiting list to attend the program.

Now diverse groups were gathering—the prosperous and poor, the educated and uninformed, the young and old, those who worked with their heads and those who worked with their hands and muscles, but that only made the experience more valuable. For people were no longer encrusted by their sameness but, rather, enlightened through their differences.

Adventures In Attitudes continued to accelerate in popularity. I did nothing to promote it. The concept was apparently encapsulated with its own nourishment. I was, in fact, somewhat a captive of this rapidly growing child. I was asked to start the program in other facilities, even other cities. A group in Hawaii transported me there to work out the mechanics for conducting the course, welcome duty in January as an escape from the harsh Minnesota winter.

In 1969 a bright, 35-year-old super-achiever, Leo Hauser, came to me. He had just sold his seat on the New York Stock Exchange. Aspiring for a business of his own directed toward personal development, he was intrigued with the "Adventures" concept.

So we formed "Personal Dynamics," a company to market Adventures In Attitudes. Leo was the president. He jumped into the training business up to his twitching ear lobes and quickly rose to be national president of the prestigious 29,000 member of the American Society for Training and Development. Leo was like a kitten in a yarn factory.

We trained thousands of others to conduct the program. It was staged in every conceivable setting—church basements, corporate training facilities, prisons, colleges, hospitals, and then into foreign countries.

It was translated into other languages and set in Braille for the sightless.

In the early 80s Personal Dynamics was acquired by the Carlson Learning Company, a division of the multi-billion dollar Carlson empire. That is home for Adventures in Attitudes today. It has touched the lives of millions throughout the world, even, most recently, Russia. In Japan alone, ignited by the vision of Sakan Yanagidaira, over 300,000 people have completed the 30-hour translated version of Adventures In Attitudes.

ATTITUDES EMPOWER

Much has been learned about life as it emerges from the cauldron of attitude exploration. Observed are the innermost thoughts and feelings of everyperson, butterflies that have sprung from mental cocoons, and spirits that have soared from minds longing to be nurtured and enlightened. Revealed are the clusters of attitudes that determine the flavors of life—the ones that are constructive and those that are destructive. Also observed are the mental struggles of people disheartened by adversity, setbacks, distress, and pain. Most certainly life contains those.

You can spend a lifetime exploring the mansions of the mind and finalize the search with the simple conclusion that your state of consciousness today determines your state of living tomorrow. Your life is shaped by your thoughts. Any thought that is held in the mind for a period of time becomes an attitude. And attitudes can empower or they can victimize. The choice is yours.

As you choose your attitudes you are essentially creating your life, your future. To evaluate the wisdom of your choices, look about you. You are looking into a mirror of your thoughts. Your life is a reflection of your attitudes.

Attitudes are causes and circumstances are effects. The daily events—the ups and downs, the bumps and bruises, the joys and festivities, and the streams of turbulance or peace—are not caused by the date on which you were born, the position of the stars, or the knobs on your head, but, rather, by the cluster of attitudes you are empowered to create.

Not I, nor anyone else, can tell you what to do with your life and its myriad of problems. I don't have those answers. Neither does your therapist, counselor, minister, bookstore, support group, or best friend. But you do. They may be locked and repressed in some remote chamber of your being. But they are there.

On that there rests the impact and wisdom of Socrates' sage advice to "know thyself." In that quest the ideas shared in this book will help. Working on the eight assignments will not only empower but will enlighten.

The assignments are simple, but not always easy. But that's life isn't it? Wouldn't it be dull if it were? The assignments are celebrations of your spiritual existence on this planet, odysseys of self-discovery! The third assignment, described in the next chapter, will help you chart that journey.

∞ PERSONAL EMPOWERMENT ∞

ASSIGNMENT NUMBER THREE

"Build Positive Attitudes"

The Dynamics of Attitudes

IT WAS 1857. Charles Dickens, a man of sparse education but
a genius-like talent, looked around and saw a world of opposites.
Flavored by his own life of hardship and sufficiency, humiliation
and respect, deprivation and plenty, he picked up his pen and wrote
the opening sentences for his *Tale of Two Cities.*

> *"It was the best of times, it was the worst of times, it was
> the age of wisdom, it was the age of foolishness, it was the
> epoch of belief, it was the epoch of incredulity, it was the sea-
> son of Light, it was the season of Darkness, it was the spring of
> hope, it was the winter of despair, we had everything before us,
> we had nothing before us."*

And so it was.

And so it is. Is the glass half full? Or is it half empty? We still
live in a world of opposites. Sickness and health, success and failure,
friend and foe, good and bad, wealth and poverty, beauty and ugli-
ness, comfort and hardship. So it goes, with all the variations
between the vice versas.

What you see is what you get. What you perceive is what you
will experience. So weigh your perceptions heavily on the side of the
positives and lightly on the side of the negatives.

Is this positive thinking? Perhaps. But let's look beyond positive thinking to the mansion in which we live—the mind. That is where we will always exist—the mansion of the mind. We have been told to build upon rock rather than sand. We will be safe, then, from the floods and winds of negative thoughts and situations.

The rock may be likened to attitudes, permanent habits of thoughts. Building on positive attitudes protects us from the shifting sands of thousands of daily thoughts and the quandary of sorting them out to decide if these are positive or negative.

That, then, is the third assignment for personal empowerment. Build positive attitudes.

Positive attitudes will infallibly create a positive mind. What can be expected? What are the empowering characteristics of a positive mind?

The positive mind looks at life as a potential rather than a struggle. It sees itself as an explorer on a grand adventure instead of a victim of circumstances.

The positive mind perceives a universe of plenty and abundance rather than scarcity and limitation. It faces adversity, chaos, or suffering still seeing hope and opportunity. It persists when confronted by obstacles, never quitting, never giving up, knowing that it can survive any ordeal in life.

The positive mind holds itself to be a miracle finding exhilaration in discovering and applying its resources. It knows that turmoil, discouragement, and pain are not realities, not truths, but only passing illusions of conditions.

The positive mind has no space for self-destructive thoughts. It embraces only its ideals, integrity, wondrous soul, and spirituality knowing that this is the "heaven within." It sees in all people that which is in itself—spiritual perfection, love, goodness—hidden, perhaps, but assuredly there.

The positive mind sees beauty and wonder in clouds sauntering along the sky with invitations to ride them, or moonbeams dancing along the ripples of the sea, or rolling plains plump with the season's festive growth. It sees the universe in a blade of grass or the infinite nature of a grain of sand.

The positive mind is the fruitage of positive attitudes. What are they? How are they built? What are their effects on our lives? Our personalities? Our relationships? Those were questions on my mind years ago when I was riding an all-night sleeper on the old Rock Island Zephyr running between Minneapolis and St. Louis. I was gathering material for my first class in attitudes.

I awoke in the middle of the night seeing mental images of charts. I sketched on paper what I envisioned.

Ah! The rippling effect of inspired moments! Those charts became benchmarks for Adventures In Attitudes. They have been reproduced millions of times, appearing in hospitals, offices, prisons, churches, schools, homes and by person-to-person in every conceivable event from prayer meetings to sales rallies to athletic events.

On the next page are the Dynamics of Attitudes with little change from my original diagrams sketched out on that night in a Pullman Berth.

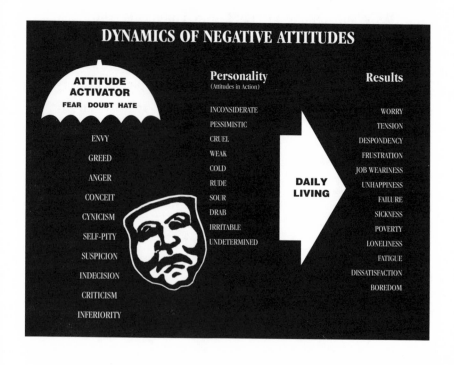

DYNAMICS OF POSITIVE ATTITUDES

UNDERSTANDING	**Personality**	**Results**
ANTICIPATION	(Attitudes in Action)	
EXPECTATIONS	ENTHUSIASTIC	SUCCESS
CONFIDENCE	DECISIVE	RECOGNITION
PATIENCE	COURAGEOUS	SECURITY
HUMILITY	OPTIMISTIC	ENERGY
BELIEF	CHEERFUL	ACHIEVEMENT
	CONSIDERATE	HAPPINESS
	FRIENDLY	GROWTH
	COURTEOUS	ADVENTURE
	SINCERE	HEALTH
	WARM	FRIENDSHIP
	RELAXED	LOVE
		INNER-PEACE

DAILY LIVING

ATTITUDE ACTIVATOR

FAITH HOPE LOVE

DYNAMICS OF NEGATIVE ATTITUDES

ATTITUDE ACTIVATOR

FEAR DOUBT HATE

	Personality	**Results**
	(Attitudes in Action)	
	INCONSIDERATE	WORRY
	PESSIMISTIC	TENSION
ENVY	CRUEL	DESPONDENCY
GREED	WEAK	FRUSTRATION
ANGER	COLD	JOB WEARINESS
CONCEIT	RUDE	UNHAPPINESS
CYNICISM	SOUR	FAILURE
SELF-PITY	DRAB	SICKNESS
SUSPICION	IRRITABLE	POVERTY
INDECISION	UNDETERMINED	LONELINESS
CRITICISM		FATIGUE
INFERIORITY		DISSATISFACTION
		BOREDOM

DAILY LIVING

A study of the charts indicates that all positive attitudes are rooted in faith, hope, or love. All negative attitudes grow out of fear, doubt, or hate. Is this a new revelation, something out of modern psychology? Hardly. It has been told by the wise and learned for centuries.

Let's go back many, many years. There was a man named Saul who was burdened with bitterness, cynicism, and prejudice. He was on his way to Damascus one day when his consciousness was jolted by the light of love. For a time he was blinded and without reason. He emerged as a transformed being, a prophet of spirituality. He became known as Paul. His words and thoughts have inspired millions for hundreds of years.

He once wrote these legendary words: "When I was a child, I spoke as a child, I understood as a child, I thought as a child: but when I became a man I put away childish things. For now we see through a glass, darkly; but then face-to-face: now I know in part; but then shall I know even as also I am known. And now abideth faith, hope, love, these three; but the greatest of these is love."

Faith, hope, love, what better rocks are there upon which to build our mansion of the mind? Develop these attitudes and there will be no room for the negatives.

Let's start with faith.

Imagine, for a moment, that you are a lonely, exhausted traveler struggling to survive on a seldom-used trail across the Amargosa Desert. Your parched throat is crying for water.

Suddenly up ahead you see an old pump. Is it a mirage? You get closer. No, it is real! Reaching out to start pumping you see a tin can wired to the handle. In it is this letter:

"This pump is all right as of June 1996. I put a new sucker washer into it and it ought to last five years but the washer

dries out and the pump has got to be primed. Under the white rock I buried a bottle of water, out of the sun and cork end up. There's enough water in it to prime the pump, but not if you drink some first. Pour about one fourth and let her soak to wet the leather. Then pour the rest medium fast and pump like crazy. You'll get water. The well has never run dry. Have faith. When you get watered up, fill the bottle and put it back like you found it for the next feller."

—*Desert Pete*

"P.S. Don't go drinking up the water first. Prime the pump with it and you'll get all you can hold."

What would you do? Drink the water or prime the pump?

Your answer could determine the degree to which you possess one of the important characteristics for personal achievement and success. That is faith.

Would you have the faith to accept the word and judgment of an unknown desert hermit? If you did you could have all the water you could possibly use and leave some for the next person, perhaps saving that person's life.

Or would the thought of doubt and self-concern control your decision? You might tell yourself the old fellow could be a little tippy in the head. Perhaps he was a joker. Maybe he had a score to settle with people and this was his way of getting even. Or the pump could have run dry or just not work any longer. How could you be sure that there was enough water to prime the pump?

You could reason that it is only "good judgment" to choose the least risky alternative.

So there you have it. That's life squeezed down to one small incident.

Have faith. Remove all negative thoughts. Take risks. Then

you will have all you can possibly use yourself and still take care of the next person.

Or let doubt, fear and self-concern rule your actions and receive only enough to barely get by and leave nothing for someone else.

Faith is trusting and believing. A set of religious beliefs are often categorized as a "faith." So when there is no belief there is no faith.

Examine the lives of all great people in history. There were tall ones, short ones, men, women, old and young—they came in various sizes and shapes and were completely different. Except for just one characteristic. They possessed faith and its companion, belief.

They believed in themselves and in a cause or purpose. And they had faith. They had faith in people, in life, in their goals and their daily activities.

When the qualities of faith and belief are understood it is apparent why they provide the personal power for achievement and success. To achieve one must be physically endowed with energy and drive. Personal motivation, confidence, enthusiasm, conviction, and vision are all essential.

Faith and belief provide these qualities.

Those who have faith and belief also build an immunity to the damaging effect of the doubters, the cynics, the complainers, the malcontents, and those who live in the shadows of pessimism.

Belief and faith! What magnificent qualities of mind that the human being can possess! They form the foundation for a life of achievement and fulfillment.

What is belief? It is the mental state of believing—a process of declaring conviction, trust, confidence, and acceptance that certain things are true and real. Belief coupled with faith transforms into unquestioning allegiance, commitment, and loyalty to something even though absolute certainty or proof may be absent.

There are some things in life deserving of that sort of mental dedication—not only deserving, they demand it. Your soul, for example, is crying out for your belief in its splendor, its integrity, its mysticism. It will return what you give it. Believe in your soul and it will return strength, miracles, character, and survival over pain and adversity.

Believe in life, for as William James advises: "Be not afraid of life; believe that life is worth living, and your belief will help create the fact."

Believe in your values. Values are the windows of the soul through which the soul can see the world and direct your intuitive instincts. Without belief, values are only whimsical notions wilting when tested.

Believe in a relationship, a family, a loved one, or just another individual. There is no greater support for rising above mediocrity and limitations than one person's belief in another.

Believe in the service you render each day—whether it is in or out of a home—no matter if you work with your head, your heart, or your muscles—believe in it. You can't do that, you say? There are too many dull, unpleasant, thankless things about what you do? For a moment, set those aside. Look for the satisfaction, fulfillment, and service in every part of your daily activity. As Goethe, the German philosopher, said, "The secret of life is not to do what you like, but to like what you do."

Believing in what you do—its purpose, its meaning—is the fountain from which enthusiasm, motivation, passion, and joy flow. Joy. That's significant. Kahlil Gibran declares:

"You work that you may keep pace with
the earth and the soul of the earth.
Work is love made visible.
And if you cannot work with love
but only with distaste, it is
better that you should leave
your work and sit at the
gate of the temple and take
alms of those who work
with joy."*

Believe in yourself. Believe in your strengths, talents, resources, and potential. You have often been compared to a snowflake—there are no two alike. You are a one-of-a-kind wonder spending a breath of time on this planet for a purpose. Believe that. Don't waste it.

Believe in your freedom. You are not free if you are obsessed with self-concern. You are not free if you are always testing the attitudes and remarks of others to determine if your own fragile self-concept has been violated. You are not free if others cannot speak spontaneously and openly of their opinions and feelings without risk of your judgment or friendship. You are not free unless you believe in your own self-worth. Does this mean that you lack humility? No. For to be free is to be humble. Humility is not being devoid of self-esteem and self-confidence. Quite the opposite. Humility is the realization of the importance of others and your eagerness and ability to serve, help, and love them. That's the humility that sets one free from one's own exalted sense of pomposity.

---

*Reprinted from *The Prophet*, by Kahlil Gibran with the permission of the publisher, Alfred A. Knopf, Inc. Copyright 1923 by Kahlil Gibran; renewal copyright 1951 by Administrators C. T. A. of Kahlil Gibran Estate and Mary G. Gibran.

There are other activities or purposes in which you may choose to believe, knowing that your belief is empowering. For "If thou canst believe, all things are possible to him that believeth." (Mark 9:23)

Which leads us to the most omnipotent of beliefs—believe in your God. Place no other beliefs before this one. Believe in the infinitude and miracle of the higher power that is the life of your life. You are not a human being seeking spirituality. You are a spiritual being dwelling in a fleshy temple of humanness. Believe in the allness of God—in you, around you, through you. This is the spiritual oneness from which you are never separate.

Dare to believe in the energy of God restoring and regenerating every cell of your body. Believe in all that God is—mercy, goodness, principle, truth, perfection, intelligence, peace, joy, love. Let your mind dwell on these things. That's the essence of a positive mind. Believe. Have faith.

Some say believing closes the mind. Not true. Believing opens the mind to unexplored depths and meanings of life. That's awareness, the awakening of your spirituality. Your birth was not the birth of your spirit, but only the birth of your awareness—a beginning of which there is no ending. You will go through levels of your awareness. When your consciousness becomes enlightened at one level you will then move on to the next level. That's life—a spiritual quest. All of your experiences, whether branded good or bad, successes or failures, joyful or painful, are only lessons on your spiritual quests—lessons to enhance your awareness.

With awareness comes enlightenment, a pathway rather than a destination that is never reached. It is a label of hope rather than an achievement. For ages humans have sought enlightenment, the divine revelation of the mystery of life. Some say it can be done in years; others claim it can be an instant unveiling. For example, Shaka, the historical founder of Buddhism in India, spent six years in the mountains to find enlightenment. He never found it, so returned to the world to seek enlightenment by other means. On the other hand, in China during the fourteenth century the central belief of the iconoclastic Chan Buddhist sect was sudden enlightenment. It was thought that this state of mind was achieved in a momentary spontaneous flash, perhaps triggered by a simple mundane act or thought.

Instant or prolonged enlightenment? The controversy will never be settled, or the term enlightenment even defined. How you perceive it is your own singular understanding. But how you achieve it can only be through awareness. And there is no awareness without belief. For belief sensitizes and awakens awareness.

Believe! Have faith!

How? How do you believe? How do you have faith? What comes first, faith or belief? It doesn't much matter. They are co-creators of your consciousness. Your mind is a disciple of your center of beliefs. In these have faith.

Believing is a mental ability, learned and developed like any other habit of thought. It starts with a decision. It can be as simple as an affirmation like this:

"In this I believe. This is my passion, my devotion, my dedication to which I am committed."

You might find it helpful to write down those things in which you believe—your values, your strengths, your spiritual convictions.

Having faith and belief implies discarding negative notions and criticisms. That would suggest that bashing the company during coffee breaks or fault-finding of another or yourself would be avoided.

You believe and have faith in that which you can demonstrate. I heard an amusing story that illustrates this sort of demonstration.

It is a fable told about the famed Zumbrati, who walked a tightrope across Niagara Falls. Conditions were less than ideal. It was a windy day. The performer was thankful to have made it across.

One of those waiting to congratulate him was a man with a wheelbarrow.

"I believe you could walk across pushing this wheelbarrow," the man told him.

Zumbrati shook his head and said he felt fortunate to have accomplished the feat without a wheelbarrow.

The man urged him to try, "I believe that you can do it," he said.

The aerialist declined, but the man kept after him.

Finally the performer said, "You really do believe in me, don't you?"

"Oh, I do," the man assured him.

"OK," Zumbrati replied. "Get in the wheelbarrow."

Get in the wheelbarrow! Demonstrate. Your beliefs are the delivery systems for your soul's expression. Commit to them. Let them be alive, seen by the world through your daily activities.

Lin Yutang, the Chinese sage, wrote: "It is not so much what you believe in that matters, as the way in which you believe, and translate that belief into action."

Faith and belief are sources of internal energy providing one with the vigor to push beyond ordinary levels of achievement.

John Stuart Mills disclosed: "One person with a belief is equal to a force of ninety-nine who only have interests."

Is there a price to be paid by believing and becoming committed to beliefs? Of course. But the price of not believing is far greater. John W. Gardner, former president of the Carnegie Corporation, once said, "The best kept secret in America today is that people would rather work hard for something they believe in than enjoy a pampered idleness. Every person knows there is exhilaration in intense effort applied toward a meaningful end."

"…be of good comfort; thy faith hath made thee whole."
—Matthew 9:22

Have faith! Believe! These are the bedrocks of positive attitudes. These are the piers upon which the positive mind is built.

Let's consider the second attribute of the positive mind—hope. Hope is a word often used lightly and loosely in daily conversation. It is, however, of profound significance in your life. Life is not always easy. There can be pain, setbacks, invalidism, and suffering. Hope is the soul's tool for enduring these adversities. As long as you have one breath of life you have cause for hope. You have something to give—a purpose and reason for being. Never ever give up hope. It is the lifeline to survival. No matter how dark or bleak or painful is the present, one faint ray of hope can be the light that removes the darkness.

Decide to believe. Have faith. Demonstrate. Get in the wheelbarrow.

Believe in the future. Leave behind the baggage and burdens of the past. Have faith that new dawns of awareness and divine vistas of bliss and peace are waiting to enhance your consciousness. For "Faith is the assurance of things hoped for, the conviction of things not seen." (Heb 11:1)

Hope. That's the second benchmark of the positive mind. Emily Dickinson adds that:

> *"Hope is the thing with feathers*
> *That perches on the soul."*

Let's consider that in the next chapter.

SEVEN

Look Up! Have Hope!

A SMALL BOY, WALKING ALONG THE SIDEWALK, SAW A BRIGHT
COPPER PENNY GLISTENING AT HIS FEET. He picked it up eagerly. He felt
a glow of pride and excitement! It was his! And it had cost him
nothing!

After that, wherever he went, he walked with his head bent
down, eyes searching the ground for more treasure. During his lifetime he found 296 pennies, 48 nickels, 19 dimes, 16 quarters, 2 half
dollars, and one crinkled paper dollar—a total of $13.26!

He got the money for nothing—except that he missed the
breathless beauty of 31,369 sunsets, the colorful splendor of 157
rainbows, the fiery brilliance of hundreds of maples nipped by the
autumn frost, white clouds drifting across the blue sky in thousands
of different billowy formations, birds flying, sun shining, and the
smiles of passing people.

How many people do you know like that, who go through
life so burdened with the trivial things that the magnificent adventure of living completely escapes them? They keep their heads bent
down looking at aches and pains, worries and fears that never happen, criticism and judgment of people, petty day-to-day problems,
and hoping to find that copper penny that they get for nothing.

If only they would look up, even for awhile and open their
minds to the unlimited dimensions of life! If they could catch a

glimpse of the boundless nature of their own inner resources they might discover the freedom, abundance, and joy that is theirs for the claiming!

Many people are so accustomed to being what they are that they are fearful of trying to be anything else. They do not hold any real hope of being anything much different from what they are. They see themselves as being trapped in a body of flesh and bones that they try to preserve for as many years as possible, frightened by the apprehension that they have very little to do with how long they last or what happens to them. They feel a burden of inadequacy, inferiority, and limitation. The things that would bring love, fulfillment, happiness, and success seem just out of reach.

The clamor of these negative sounds seems to hammer people into a submissive state of mind in which they exist for a lifetime overpowered by feelings of despair, discouragement, helplessness, and doubt. They hang on to their negative attitudes, guarding them tenaciously as being reality. In fact, it has been found that people tend to protect their negative mind-sets more vigorously than the positive ones.

In Russia many years ago a Czar came upon a sentry standing at attention in a secluded spot in the palace garden. He asked the man, "Sentry, what are you guarding?"

"I don't know, Sire," the guard replied. "I was ordered to my post by the Captain of the Guard."

Calling the Captain of the Guard, the Czar questioned him concerning the sentry's post. The Captain could give no better answer than, "Regulations call for a sentry at that particular spot."

Determined to find the reason for this apparently useless provision, the Czar ordered the archives to be searched to determine the origin of the regulation. Finally it was learned that many years before, Catherine the Great had planted a rose bush there and ordered a sentry placed beside it to keep it from being trampled. The rose bush had been dead over one hundred years, but the sentry was still there.

Many people are standing guard over rose bushes in the mind—phantoms of the past that restrain and hold them back. Misery, woe, misfortune, doubt, pessimism, and cynicism are all burdensome rose bushes that can be set aside by replacing them with hope, the second footing upon which the positive mind is built. A mind focusing on hope will crowd out worry and pain and fear. Hope is the light of the soul giving it freedom and nourishment for growth and expression.

Hope is knowing that there is a divine presence unfolding in your life with a singular plan for a splendid purpose. You have a supreme possibility within your being, a seed of greatness, an undiscovered potential resting within. Hope will awaken that capacity.

Hope is not cloned by human nature. It is chosen. It is created by one of the most wondrous mechanisms in the universe—your imagination. No other form of life has that. In your imagination you can envision, expect, hope, and create pictures of the future that exhilarate and excite. That's hope. And what you envision and hope for you will most likely experience whether it's finding a four leaf clover or a dinosaur egg in the Gobi desert. Hope invigorates, enthuses; it is the whip that drives the emotions—the fuel of desire.

Yes, life should be lived in the now. But the now can be ever more joyful if filled with hope. Hope, after all, shapes tomorrow's now. And what is "now"? Now is yesterday's future—yesterday's hope arrived.

It is nurturing and enchanting to use the imaginary senses to look ahead, to expect miracles. That's hope. Envision dancing with blissful moments, weeping with episodes of joy, walking with the tempo of tomorrow's activities, breathing with the ecstasy of the wind, the rain, the sunshine.

Hope is also, as John Stuart Mills suggests, "...best to remember that life is not a judgment to drudgery. It is glory, a dignity, an opportunity, a prelude, and a reward. The true life has a deep content in itself, in its worlds, in its brotherhood. It is to play, to rejoice with the hills, to throb with the sea, to laugh with nature, as well as to struggle and pile up victories."

Hope is the elixir of the mind, the stuff from which dreams are built.

HAVE A DREAM

If you look to a dream, nurture it, and hold it close to your heart, then what you see, you will most certainly experience!

Your dreams are the wings of your thoughts; they lift your thinking out of the commonplace and ordinary. Belief and dedication motivate, but dreams inspire!

Your dreams of tomorrow will make today's problems seem unimportant—the crumbs on the floor, the worn-out tire, the corn on the toe, the complaints of customers, and the dreary turn-downs will fall from your thoughts like dried leaves from a tree if you have a big dream.

Dreams take the dullness out of work, the aggravation from problems, and the hopelessness from lack. They are the cups that hold your efforts. Your cup will truly "runneth over" with your dreams fulfilled unless you let others punch holes in it!

Hold fast to your dreams! They are the harps of the heart that add music to your everyday existence!

In the 1800's James Allen wrote:

"The dreamers are the saviors of the world.

"Humanity cannot forget its dreamers; it cannot let their trials fade and die; it lives in them; it knows them as the realities which it shall one day see and know.

"Cherish your visions; cherish your ideals; cherish the music that stirs in your heart, the beauty that forms in your mind, the loveliness that drapes your purest thoughts. Out of them will grow all delightful conditions, all heavenly environment. Of them, if you but remain true to them, your world will at last be built.

"Dream lofty dreams, and as you dream, so shall you become."

Modern psychologists have done little but reaffirm Allen's intuitive philosophies. James Garfield, president of Performance Sciences Institute, spent two decades studying the characteristics of 1,500 super-achievers.

Peak performance, he found, begins with a mission. Without a dream, a compelling inner urge life becomes a workaday routine. And that is acceptable for many, but not the dreamers.

Having a dream and then having the tenacity to stick to it longer than anyone else is more important to success than innate ability or raw talent, Garfield reports.

What he doesn't say is that dreamers have little choice except to abide with their visions. For the dreamers, you see, do not know how to give up. That's right. They literally do not know how to give up. They know how to plod, grub, sacrifice, grind and strive, but they do not know how to give up.

Failure does not occur to the visionary. The efforts, trials, futilities and methods might fail, but not the dreams. In fact, failure endows to the dreamer a sense of exhilaration as if it were a stepping stone towards the realization of the goal.

Thomas Edison expressed this once when asked, "Mr. Edison, you have failed over 1,000 times in your attempt to develop a filament for the light bulb. When are you going to give up or stop trying?"

"I haven't failed 1,000 times," the inventor replied. "I've only discovered a thousand ways it can't be done."

That is somewhat like the small boy playing sandlot baseball.

His father came by and called out, "How are you doing, Tommy? What's the score?"

"Nineteen to nothing," the boy replied.

"Whose favor?" asked Dad.

"Theirs!" was the response.

"You're really being clobbered, aren't you, Tommy?" cried the father.

"Shucks no, Dad. We ain't even been to bat yet!" answered Tommy.

So, a dream reduces the day's obstacles and setbacks to insignificance. When many are driven to sleepless nights and knotted stomachs by reverses and hardships, the dreamer is at peace. The rainbows and mountain tops rest within the soul of the dreamer. The crevices and boulders are only adornments along the way to the vision.

A dreamer is little concerned with details or methods. Let others become ensnared with those. A dreamer knows there are many pathways to a destination. If one leads to a dead end, then another will be found.

Dreamers do not necessarily follow the paths of others. They go, instead, where there is no path and leave a trail.

To the person who aspires toward a vision, each day is more elevated than the one before. It is this knowingness in the heart of the dreamer that makes life a constant ascendancy toward the stars.

Dreams are like those stars. They will never be touched, but they become guides in darkness. Following them will ensure that one's destiny will be reached.

Henry David Thoreau would agree. From the edge of Walden Pond he wrote: "If one advances confidently in the direction of one's dreams, and endeavors to live the life that is imagined, one will meet with a success unexpected in common hours."

So find a dream. Keep it, nurture it, hold it close to your heart. To let it go is to die; your spirit shrivels.

Dreams enthuse; they erase dullness from your life. Verily they become life itself.

SET GOALS

Dreams must inevitably lead to specific goals. Dreams are the visions; goals become the plans by which dreams materialize.

A ship without a pilot or course would drift aimlessly about the sea, being driven by the waves and wind, eventually ending up a wreck on some barren shore.

A human life is not much different. Without direction and purpose and a mind firmly in control, fate and circumstances alone will determine one's destiny.

No individual need sacrifice one's life to such chance and happenstance, however. For the human being, apart from all other forms of life, is given the power to choose the paths of existence.

Journeys through life can be charted, planned and experienced by the intellect and will of the individual. The process begins with setting destinations or goals. That is apparently life's ultimate purpose.

Goals shape people's lives. They determine the courses of people's destinies, molding circumstances, and eventually, the inner characteristics of attitude, thought, and feeling. People are exactly where they choose to be because of their goals. A vagrant wanders about the street, penniless, seeking only food and a place to sleep. Those have become the only daily goals. Not lofty goals, of course, but goals nonetheless.

People's everyday existence is regulated by their goals. They start living by goals very early in life. Usually their parents started setting their goals for them. Go to school. Work hard. Be good. Get a job. Such fundamentals were implanted as goals in the minds of most at a very early age. They have never changed.

Along the way, however, many pick up other goals. Impress others. Watch TV. Socialize. Take things easy. Avoid failure. Don't get involved with too many things. Look around for ways to make more money. Change jobs. Spend time with family or friends. Get a hobby.

The list is endless. In fact, it is so long that goals become the primary source of conflict and frustration in people's lives.

You know people who are chasing from morning 'til night, busy as kittens in a yarn basket and not accomplishing much more. Each task, each errand, started as a deliberately chosen goal, eventually becoming a series of habits. Confusion and chaos are then a way of life.

All of these lives could be lifted from mediocrity by following the advice of Frank Lloyd Wright, the famed American architect. He is credited with saying, "Make no little plans, for there is no magic in them to stir people's souls."

His plans were blueprints that started as dreams. Then his dreams became goals. So make no little goals, for there is no energy in them to empower you to the larger dimensions of life. Most people are letting dozens and dozens of trivial goals and habits dominate their day-to-day lives. Where they will be five and ten years from now is simply an extension of where they are today.

If you would dare break out of self-imposed boundaries, set goals. They can be realistic and achievable as long as they are constantly progressing. As one level is realized, another a bit higher is then established.

That is the thrill and excitement of the unlimited nature of life—always reaching out and achieving a new and higher goal. That is also the only way to discover the invisible greatness within you.

Many people won't admit that exists. They see themselves as quite average and not rising much above what they are now.

People have been found to set goals to match their self-images. If they see themselves as mediocre, they set mediocre goals. They will then do as little or as much as they must do to meet their goals and preserve their self-images.

Forget about what you have done or holding yourself back when setting goals.

It is always amazing to witness the transformation in people's lives when they learn how to use goals. For a goal held in the mind, nurtured and stimulated by desire, will inevitably change the person.

New talents, unknown abilities, and fresh enthusiasm will blossom from a mind opened by the pursuit of a goal. The person will excitedly proclaim, "I have discovered I can do something I never knew I could do before."

The individual will have been awakened by a newfound power that need never be exhausted as the boundless potentials of life are explored. This process, be assured, is not fantasy or motivational vaccination. Experiences like this are well-documented events that have occurred in the lives of people like yourself.

It starts in the human mind with a determination to "make no little plans."

Those might sound like story book words. But silence your skepticism for a moment.

Dare to believe you can unfasten the chains that have held you back from a life that you have only dreamed possible. For you to suppose you have to travel a long distance to get where you want to go is false. You must trust that you are already there. That is the essence of hope laced with belief.

So drench your mind with the forces of hope. Look up! Surrender and connect! Expect miracles! Believe! Dream! Set goals!

Faith, hope, and love. Those are the pillars upon which positive attitudes are built. We have considered faith and hope. Let's look at love.

If you look earnestly and honestly into the depths of your heart you might find clouds of doubt and futility obscuring your ability to love, especially…

If you have loved and loved, only to feel your love meant little to others…

Or if you have loved with all the energy your soul could muster only to have that love twisted and wrenched by another…

Or if you want to love but can find no one to love…

Or if you are attacked by others who may threaten your integrity or self-esteem and are told you should love them but feel that you can't…

Or if you see others hugging and embracing but feel strangeness about doing that yourself…

Or if it seems that everyone around you is having a banquet of love but you haven't been invited…

Or if you have heard of the wonders and joys of love but are still searching for them yourself…

Or if you find yourself being critical of some of those who talk about love…

Or if you have to make decisions that are anything but loving…

Or if you find that you get angry or upset with those you are supposed to love…

Or if you must disentangle your life from the lives of others because of their self-inflicted misery and despair and then be accused of not loving…

Or if you have been endowed with power or authority over others and must treat their indifference or incompetence with logic rather than love…

Or if you have been abused physically or emotionally by another and find it quite impossible to replace resentment with love…

Or if you have been told to love your enemies and have tried and tried but somehow can't…

Or if you know people who are glowing with love and you long to be like them but feel you never will be…

Or if there are those who are treating you unfairly but forgiveness is stuck in your heart and will not let you love…

Or if there are those in your life who, by marriage or family relationship, you know you should love, but the feeling just is not there…

If you have had any of these feelings and sense a hardening of your heart, a hovering coldness toward some, a gnawing guilt about not loving, or have been told that "God is love" and your unloving makes you feel apart from God, then come along with me for the next two chapters; we'll toss around some ideas about life and love and why you should not spend another moment feeling that you are anything other than a wondrous human being whose life can be fuller and richer by understanding love and be empowered by the energy of love.

⮺ PERSONAL EMPOWERMENT ⮺

ASSIGNMENT NUMBER FOUR

"Love Unconditionally"

EIGHT

Lessons in Love

*Though I speak with the tongues of men and of
angels, and have not Love, I am become as sounding
brass, or a tinkling cymbal. And though I have the
gift of prophecy, and understanding all mysteries, and
all knowledge; and though I have all faith, so that I
could remove mountains, and have not Love, I am
nothing. And though I bestow all my goods to feed the
poor, and though I give my body to be burned, and
have not Love, it profiteth me nothing. Love suffereth
long, and is kind; Love envieth not; Love vaunteth not
itself, is not puffed up, Doth not behave itself unseemly,
Seeketh not her own, Is not easily provoked, Thinketh
no evil; Rejoiceth not in iniquity, but rejoiceth in the
truth; Beareth all things, believeth all things, hopeth
all things, endureth all things.*

*Love never faileth: but whether there be
prophecies, they shall fail; whether there be tongues,
they shall cease; whether there be knowledge, it shall
vanish away. For we know in part, and we prophesy in
part. But when that which is perfect is come, then that
which is in part shall be done away. When I was a
child, I spake as a child, I understood as a child, I
thought as a child: but when I became a man I put
away childish things. For now we see through a glass,*

*darkly; but then face to face: now I know in part; but
then shall I know even as also I am known. And now
abideth faith, hope, Love, these three; but the greatest
of these is Love.*

—*I Cor. 13.*

THE LIGHT OF LOVE

Love works; hate doesn't.

Love makes your life better; hate does quite the opposite.

Hate has many shadows—prejudice, resentment, sarcasm, racism, bias, envy, brutality, discrimination, revenge, caustic criticism.

Love nurtures; hate suffocates.

Love heals; hate sickens.

Love frees; hate enslaves.

Love unifies; hate divides.

Love strengthens; hate weakens.

Love attracts; hate repels.

Love restores; hate erodes.

Love comforts; hate distresses.

Love is beautiful; hate is ugly.

Love is an asset; hate is a liability.

Love is cheer; hate is gloom.

Love is harmony; hate is discord.

Love is boundless; hate is restricting.

Love is faith; hate is fear.

Love is friendship; hate is loneliness.

Love is constructive; hate is destructive.

Love is fulfillment; hate is emptiness.

Love is joy; hate is despair.

Love is wisdom; hate is ignorance.

Love is peace; hate is hostility.

Love is hope; hate is doubt.

Love empowers; hate, with all its cannibalistic appetites, will devour your wholeness.

It should come as no surprise that the fourth assignment for personal empowerment is "Love Unconditionally."

We are here to express love, that comes before all else.

The word "love" is used in so many different ways that we become confused about its meaning. You are told, for example, to "love your neighbor."

"Love my neighbor?" you ask. "Those people whose stereo and parties keep me awake at night? Whose kids torment mine? Whose dog dirties my lawn? Love them? We aren't even speaking to each other!"

There are times you can't always love with people pushing, crowding, and taking advantage of you. There are those who would cheat you, take what is yours, ignore you, and cause pain and suffer-ing—even those whom you expect to love you.

Besides, there are unruly children, goof-offs at work, and overbearing relatives all causing irritation, aggravation, and frustra-tion—certainly not love. So you feel unloving. Loving uncondition-ally is beyond you.

And that creates guilt; the dictum to "love unconditionally" lays a lot of guilt on a lot of people. There are women, for instance, who actually believe they deserve physical abuse from brutes who con-vince the distraught ladies that they aren't as loving as they should be.

With guilt comes a loss of self-esteem. If you can't love oth-ers how can you love yourself?

Love should not be a boomerang that brings back heartache and remorse. Love is joy, fulfillment, and empowerment.

Understanding what it is and how to do it may make it more natural and easy to "love unconditionally."

What Is Love?

Let's set aside the mind-set that love is a feeling. Love is thinking and doing. It starts out as an attitude and ends up as a feeling. Many try to reverse that. They search frantically for the rapture of love, expecting it to fill their minds with blissful thoughts. It seldom happens. There are too many people, also, who are looking for love in sex, drugs, and frizzly attachments and ending up in a cactus patch. Don't put yourself on that shelf. Think of love as an attitude. That is the root. The feeling of love is the growth, the blossom.

The fact that you do not have a feeling of love does not mean that you do not love unconditionally. In realizing that love is an attitude, there are many ways to love unconditionally that are simply thinking and doing.

You can, for instance, be kind. The world reveres kindness. It is a dear quality that gives warmth and gratitude to others.

You see an individual helping a sightless person across the street. A woman cooks a warm meal for the neighboring family of a sick mother. A boy picks the burrs from the hair of a stray dog. A farmer takes in and cares for a motherless fawn.

These are acts of kindness. The list is endless. The consequences are always the same—admiration, feelings of friendliness, esteem, affection.

In modern times there are so many detours from kindness. The high standards of living that breed indifference, the pressures of mass production, the echelons of authority, and the general hurry-scurry that exist all seem to be shoving kindness aside—making it a neglected virtue.

But this makes it an even more precious and valued attribute. Its scarcity renders it ever more powerful!

How do you get it? How do you become a "kind" person? To develop qualities of kindness you would learn from one who is kind.

Along with Mother Theresa, one of the most humane people of modern times would be Dr. Albert Schweitzer.

At the age of 38, Dr. Schweitzer forsook all of the comforts and conveniences his great genius could provide in the civilized world. He went to the uncivilized, hot steaming jungle in what was then French Equatorial Africa. He built a hospital in Lambarene near Gabon.

There he surrounded himself with life in all forms—monkeys, dogs, cats, goats, sheep, antelopes, owls, pelicans, and storks, to name a few. And there life was truly respected and treated kindly. The natives were ministered to for their sickness and disease. The animals were cared for. Nothing was maliciously killed.

How could one who respected life so deeply be anything but kind?

Dr. Schweitzer once wrote:

"Our civilization lacks human feeling. We are humans who are insufficiently humane! We must realize and seek to find a new spirit. We have lost sight of this ideal because we are solely occupied with thoughts of people, instead of remembering that our goodness and compassion should extend to all life."

Kindness is a response to pain, suffering, and the problems of life.

Eliminate any thought that kindness is a "do-gooder" trait reserved for those who have nothing better to do. Or that it is a trait of the weak who are afraid to do anything wrong and therefore end up being kind.

Kindness is a strong, respected quality. It requires a willingness to give some measure of one's self for the benefit of others. And that, perhaps, is the feature of kindness that has made it such a compelling influence among people. It is a reflection of the time-honored dictate: "Love thy neighbor."

LOVE IS UNDERSTANDING

You have probably heard someone say, "Thank you for your love and understanding." Love, understanding. They seem to be companions. Let's take a closer look.

You've just gotten into a new car at the dealer's. You start the motor. It purrs, scarcely audible. You coast on to the road. You head toward home with this factory-fresh, spotless beauty.

There's a small boy ahead on the side of the road. Is he going to cross over? You slow down. As you pass him you hear a thud on the side of the car. That little rascal threw something to scar the glistening panel. You stop the car and look back. The boy is still there.

What kind of little monster is he? He can't be over seven or eight. He's got a lot to learn, beginning right now. What kind of parents would raise a boy like that? You're about to find out because that's where you're going to trundle him. The brand new car marred before you even got home! With each step the blood pressure and anger go up a few notches.

You walk up to him, look down, and get ready to unload. Then a cherub-like face looks up and panicky words blurt out. "I was sorry to do that but it was the only way I knew to stop your car. My little brother has been hurt real bad. Would you help him? Please?"

What happens to the anger? The judgment? The punishment? Chances are the emotions have melted and been replaced by understanding. Now you understand why the boy acted the way he did. With understanding comes caring, compassion, and an impulse to help. And that's love.

Understanding is reaching out to others, putting yourself in their shoes, knowing that they do things for their reasons, not yours. You seldom know what those reasons are, even if you were Sigmund Freud or Carl Jung. You don't always understand yourself. How can you understand others?

But you can communicate understanding. Don't judge. Be tolerant. Listen. Show interest, compassion, kindness. Above all, do not withhold your love just because you do not understand what is behind the words and actions of others. If you do you're going to be holding back a heap of love that could be out there doing a lot of good, empowering you.

Admittedly there is a tendency to do just that. We apparently have a burr in our underthings that keeps jabbing us to try to understand the behavior of others, especially those closest to us. We have an unsatisfied urge to understand.

"Why do you act that way?"

"Why in the world would he do such a thing?"

"What makes you say things like that?"

"I want to know what's going on here."

It goes deeper. So we read books, go to seminars, get in line for the therapist, and join support groups. Is it all for naught? Of course not. It's a way of growing, part of the enchantment of life. But unless we recognize the evasive nature of understanding, we're apt to get caught in its sneaky undertow. For, you see, we fear that which we do not understand. And when we don't understand the behavior of others or their feelings for us then fear creeps in. And that obstructs love.

That's when we must remind ourselves to love unconditionally. Don't make it necessary for the boy to explain why he threw the object at the car before you start loving him. Don't require people to change to your understanding to receive your love. Don't demand that they explain themselves so that you can love them.

Just love unconditionally. Be tolerant, accepting, compassionate, and kind. That's what unconditional love is. That's also understanding.

Loving Is Giving

There is one more characteristic of unconditional love that is empowering. By giving we receive. Only by forgetting ourselves are we remembered. When giving ourselves away, we find ourselves. By acts of love we surrender the burdens we have gathered.

That is taught in an old Chinese tale about a woman whose only son died. In distress she went to a holy man and pleaded, "What mystic powers do you have that will lift the ache from my heart?"

Rather than reason with her he said, "Fetch me a mustard seed from a home that has never known sorrow. We will use it to drive the pain from your life." The woman set out in search for the miracle seed.

She approached a stately mansion, knocked on the door, and asked, "I am seeking a home that has never known sadness. Is this such a place?"

"You have come to the wrong home," she was told. Then followed a description of tragedy and hopelessness that had befallen the residents.

The woman thought to herself, "Who is more able to help these desperate people than myself who has also known such pain?" So she stayed and comforted them.

She went on, seeking a home that had never known sorrow. But wherever she went, from the simplest to the grandest of lodgings, she found stories of suffering and misfortune. In each instance, she stayed long enough to share and minister to the other people's grief.

In so doing, she forgot about her quest for the magical mustard seed, never realizing it had, in fact, driven the sorrow out of her life.

So, we are reminded that we often find what we want only when we stop looking. Our focus must be on others' wants rather than our own.

Albert Einstein said it this way:

"Strange is our situation here upon earth. Each of us comes for a short visit, not knowing why, yet sometimes seeming to a divine purpose.

"From the standpoint of daily life, however, there is one thing we do know: That we are here for the sake of others…for the countless unknown souls with whose fate we are connected by a bond of sympathy.

"Many times a day I realize how much my own outer and inner life is built upon the labors of people, both living and dead, and how earnestly I must exert myself in order to give in return as much as I have received."

Such giving is often confused with loss. Erich Fromm reshapes this distortion:

"The most widespread misunderstanding is that giving is 'giving up' something, being deprived of, sacrificing. People feel giving is an impoverishment…In the very act of giving I experience my strength, my wealth, my power. This experience of heightened vitality and potency fills me with joy. I experience myself as overflowing, spending, alive, hence as joyous. Giving is more joyous than receiving, not because it is a deprivation, but because in the act of giving lies the expression of my aliveness."

So loving unconditionally is simply giving of yourself without conditions and expectations. There are those who place conditions on their love. They're saying:

"I'll love you if you'll love me."

"You would be a lot more lovable if you'd quit complaining."

"If you weighed less or dressed differently I'd love you more."

"How can I love you when you act that way?"

"Work harder, be nicer, smile, clean your room, talk to me, stop smoking, get a different job, remember my birthday, treat me better, think of someone besides yourself, be what I think you should be then I'll give you my love."

"Besides that if you don't phone once in a while, or say 'thank you' when I give you something, or write when I write, or invite me over you won't hear from me any more."

That's love withheld—easy to justify but not unconditional love. Nor does it make anyone's life any better. There are those who are holding back their love to "teach someone a lesson." How futile!

They don't seem to realize that what they are doing to others they are really doing to themselves. Love withheld is self-inflicted pain.

Look beyond the actions and behavior of others and care for them. Loving should not be dependent on the way another treats you. Just love.

In Japan, tucked high in the mountains, is an area known as "The Place Where You Leave Your Mother." Centuries ago it was believed that the old and feeble were taken there and left to die. The story is told about the strong young son carrying a frail small mother up the mountains to leave her there. He noticed that she wanted to stop frequently. Each time she would gather some sticks and break them.

Finally, he asked, "Why, Mother, do you leave a trail of broken sticks?"

"So you won't lose your way coming back, my son," replied the mother.

It is a fable of love, a mother's love. That is loving unconditionally. It is a gift of the spirit, a potential of every individual. In the days ahead, practice loving to help others find their ways. Your acts of love, like broken sticks, can provide guidance for others. Give your love without thought of what you will be getting in return. Love unconditionally.

Loving unconditionally is a field of dreams; every time it is held back an acre or two is lost.

We have put a prism to loving unconditionally and fractured it into its various colors. Show kindness, tolerance, and understanding. Give of yourself. Be non-resistant.

By becoming better acquainted with loving unconditionally you become aware that you don't have to be anyone different from who are to do it. You don't have to forsake all, go far away, meditate cross-legged in a cave, or look any further than right where you are.

To love unconditionally it is not necessary to change your feelings, just your attitudes. You don't even have to like or approve of others to love them. Nor must they alter their ways to be loved by you.

You hopefully realize now that loving unconditionally describes a large part of what you are and have been doing.

But we can all become better at it, can't we? And the better we become the more empowered we become. How do we do that? The same way we become better at anything. Practice.

Loving unconditionally is an ability that is enhanced by practice but not just random effort. Guidelines and practice techniques are needed for progressive fulfillment.

Let's work on that in the next chapter.

NINE

The Ways of Love

"How do I love thee? Let me count the ways. I love
thee to the depth and breadth and height, My
soul can reach, when feeling out of sight
for the ends of being and ideal grace."
—*Elizabeth Barrett Browning*

THINK LOVE.

Saturate your mind with the word "love."

When you're cut off in traffic—think love.

When you get a rent increase—think love.

When you're put down by another—think love.

When you give and receive nothing in return—think love.

When you're concerned about what lies ahead—think love.

When you've been cast aside in a relationship—think love.

When you're over-worked and underpaid—think love.

When you're not getting the gratitude you deserve—think love.

When someone else has been chosen instead of you—think love.

When your feelings have been scarred—think love.

When you're brushed aside with indifference—think love.

When you're in pain—think love.

When you're lonely and friendless—think love.

When it seems that the world has turned against you—think love.

When you're upset with someone close to you—think love.

Look into the troubled eyes of a stranger and think love.

If you are impatient with the driver ahead of you, or the person serving your lunch is inept, or the one checking out groceries is discourteous, or someone crowds in ahead of you—think love.

Think love.

That is the first of five rules for practicing to love unconditionally; for learning to love.

Think love. It seems simple, but it's not always easy. Loving unconditionally goes deeper, becomes more difficult.

You are threatened, intimidated, cheated, or treated harshly—think love. Remember, you don't have to change your mind or behavior. Just think love. Say it to yourself—love, love, love. Repeat it over and over. You can do that, can't you?

When you learn about those who break the law, think love.

When you see the homeless and unlovable, think love.

When you read about the juveniles and their gangs, drugs, and lovelessness, think love.

It won't work, you might think. It doesn't make you or them any better. Doesn't it?

Meet Jim Beattie. Or, perhaps you have if you're a classic movie buff. He was an aspiring actor who played the title role in *The Great White Hope*. Jim, 6'9", lanky, muscular, and ruggedly attractive, was a nationally ranked boxer at the time. He had only to be himself in the role of the pugilist in the film.

Swayed by public adoration, money, and the corruptive pressures of the fight business, Beattie became entangled with drugs and the wrong kind of people. He pulled the reins on himself before it was too late and entered a corrective facility. He came out clean.

Jim also nurtured a vision. He wanted to do for others what had been done for him. His life had suddenly been turned around by being loved rather than condemned. Could young lives in more serious trouble be transformed in the same way? By thinking love?

In the mid-1970s, Jim came to me with his dream—a two-year, live-in, therapeutic program for young felons. It would be an alternative to prison. We became committed to the project and to each other.

The obstacles were monstrous. Credibility had to be established with courts and judges. Neighborhoods were hostile toward having young criminals housed close by. Money was practically impossible to raise. Provide funds to rehabilitate felons with tough love? No siree! Lock 'em up. Punish them. Get 'em off the street.

We persisted, finally getting a toehold and a few wayward youths lodged in an abandoned building. It was named Nexus. The building was soon condemned. But not the dream.

At a snail's pace, we crept ahead, dealing with problems of people, money, and young lives that had known only abuse, brutality, addiction—never love. Staying in existence was a daily challenge.

But then came a few successes—lives saved from crime, violence, and craziness. That was twenty years ago.

Today, Nexus is the paragon of such institutions with three academies on campus-like settings. The dormitories, classrooms, recreational facilities, and therapeutic sanctums are staffed by 400 psychologists, teachers, counselors, therapists and support personnel. They are providing every day what 250 boys and girls from 6 to 18 have never received—love. In fact, most have experienced just the opposite—abuse—sexual, in some cases, which has caused their young lives to become distorted, troubled, hostile, anti-social. The Nexus dream is to save those lives from being trashed.

Have there been failures? Yes. But a multitude of heart-warming successes have kept the dream alive and growing. Am I suggesting that programs like Nexus are the answers to all of our problems of drugs, crime, violence, and brutality? Of course not. All I am proposing is to think love in every human circumstance. Unconditional love. Tough love, perhaps, but love. Hate hasn't worked. Let's try love. It won't change the world but it will work for you.

Thinking love will quiet stress and aggravation. It will mold non-resistance and deaden the spontaneous impulse to attack and defend. It will ensure sanity and reason for your human relationships.

SPEAK LOVE

The second rule to practice unconditional love is to speak love. These are the sounds of love.

I'll do that for you.

I'm proud of you.

Tell me more about what you do.

We need you.

You don't have to explain.

Take care, special person.

You have a lot to offer.

I love you.

You look wonderful.

Thank you for coming.

This flower is for you.

Let me help you.

Pardon me.

I always enjoy being with you.

You've been a big help.

I would like to know you better.

I love you.

Please.

It's my fault.

Have a nice day.

Your friendship means a lot.

Is there anything I can do for you?

Thank you.

I understand how you feel.

I love you.

Here's a book you might like.

I've been thinking about you.

Let's talk about it.

I celebrate your success.

I appreciate your thoughtfulness.

I called to see how you are.

I couldn't have done it without you.

Are you comfortable?

That's kind of you to say that.

I'm sorry.

That's no problem. I'll take care of it.

I love you.

Just keep on being who you are.

You're important.

We're better because of you.

That was a nice thing you did.

I love you.

Speak love. Thoughts of love have little meaning unless they become sounds of love. And acts of love. That, then, is the third rule for loving unconditionally. Act love.

ACT LOVE

All about you, every day, are opportunities to give meaning to your thoughts and words of love, not with the attempt to get something from others but to share what you are with them.

Act love. Give yourself away. There was a book written about that once. The author, David Dunn, gave an idea to the New York Central Railroad that was used on their advertising calendar in 1924. The only reward was seeing his brainchild come to life wherever he went.

He tried giving away his thoughts and ideas in other ways and found, always, a glow of pleasure, "A happier way of living which all so earnestly seek and so few seem to find."

His story was printed first by *Forbes*, then *Reader's Digest*, and finally put into book form under the title *Try Giving Yourself Away*.

The philosophy is simple. Let no charitable urge go unexpressed. Share your kindness, thoughtfulness, and love with others—not your money—but the little deeds that cost nothing and benefit others in some way. Expect nothing in return, not even a response.

He tells of a lot of his own experiences. Sending a picture, poem, or cartoon that would interest a friend. Buying a couple youngsters, who are standing hungrily in front of the popcorn wagon, some bags of hot, buttered popcorn. Writing letters to those who had given him attentive service. Phoning people to pay them compliments. Giving of himself became a style of thought and action that, he discovered, added a significant richness to his life.

A holiness is absorbed in acts of love, giving of yourself, expecting nothing in return. There is a Jewish story of two brothers whose farms lay side by side. One night, after the gathering of the harvest, the elder brother said to his wife, "My brother is a lonely man who has neither wife nor children. I will carry some of my sheaves into his field." But to his amazement, the next morning his stack of grain was as large as before. He continued to carry part of his harvest to his brother's farm each night, but every morning his own store of grain seemed untouched. The mystery was not revealed until one moonlit night the brothers, with their arms full of sheaves, met midway, face to face! Because of the generosity shown by the brothers, on this spot a temple was built, for the neighbors considered it to be the place where earth was nearest to heaven.

You will benefit from doing random deeds of goodness during the day. At night when you put yourself to rest you just feel good, you like yourself. It has been a day fully lived. Perhaps Mary Ann Evans, better known as George Elliot, was aware of this when she wrote:

> *If you sit down at set of sun*
> *And count the acts that you have done,*
> *And, counting, find*
> *One self-denying deed, one word*
> *That eased the heart of him who heard,*
> *One glance most kind*
> *That fell like sunshine where it went—*
> *Then you may count that day well spent.*

That leads us to the fourth rule for practicing unconditional love. Forgive.

The Power of Forgiving

We are born into a world that is unfair. It is not fair that they have earthquakes in Tokyo, floods in Iowa, hurricanes in the Caribbean, and mud slides in California. It is unfair that lions eat rabbits, unfriendly germs attack our bodies, and bad things happen to good people.

Children, playing together, react to a fracas by crying out, "That's not fair." Sibling rivalry often sparks the complaint, "You get to do that and I don't. That's not fair."

The children grow up and find the adult world not much different. People treat each other unfairly. Feelings are bruised in the workplace by favoritism and discrimination. Petty family squabbles can produce major rifts, each one claiming the other acted "unfairly."

One of the most famous short stories ever written deals with being judged unfairly. Guy de Maupassant's masterpiece *A Piece of String* tells of a Norman peasant, Master Hauchecorne, who was destroyed by his reaction to injustice.

The thirty-year-old man was walking through the bustling marketplace one day when he saw a piece of string on the ground. He stooped down, picked up the string, and put it in his pocket. He was seen doing it and was accused later of having found a wallet lost at about the same spot.

He protested vigorously but was nevertheless taken to the local police station. He displayed his piece of string but was still not believed.

The next day the wallet was found. Hauchecorne rushed to town to profess his innocence. Still he found none who would believe him.

We will let the story tell the rest.

"The peasant was thunderstruck. He understood at last. It

was insinuated that he had caused the pocketbook to be taken by someone else, an accomplice.

"He returned home, ashamed and indignant, choking with anger and bewilderment. He realized confusedly that it would be impossible to prove his innocence. And he felt wounded to the heart by the injustice of this suspicion.

"Then he began again to tell his story, making the tale a little longer every day, adding new reasons every time, more energetic protestations, most solemn oaths which he thought out and prepared in his solitary moments, for his mind was solely occupied by the story of the piece of string. They believed him less and less as his defense became more and more elaborate, his arguments more subtle.

"He was conscious of all this, but went on eating his heart out, exhausting himself in fruitless efforts.

"Before the very eyes of people, he wasted away.

"Jokers now would make him tell them about the piece of string to amuse them, as one makes old soldiers tell about their battles. His spirit, undetermined, grew feebler and feebler.

"Toward the end of December he took to his bed.

"He died at the beginning of January, and in his last delirium still protested his innocence, repeating:

"A little piece of string…a little piece of string…look, here it is, M. le Maire!"

Research indicates that the story could very well be based on fact. According to one report, the surging devastation of harbored resentment and hatred can actually kill a person. Not being able to "forgive and forget" causes the blood to clot more quickly, blood cells to increase, and stomach muscles to squeeze down and inhibit the digestive process. The overpowering effect of this intense emotion has been known to cause a stroke or heart attack.

How many "pieces of string" cause lengthy periods of suffering, anger, and mental anguish in people's lives? Insinuations, flimsy implications, and self-serving blame can trigger grudges, separation, and heartache.

The French peasant, Master Hauchecorne, acted quite naturally. Attack and defend. It brought him nothing, however, except endless misery and ultimately death.

There would have been a better response, one that would have healed his anguish. Forgiveness. Forgive those who treated him unjustly. It is as appropriate today in every human conflict as it would have been for the French peasant.

There can be no peace, no comfort, no wholeness, no love without forgiveness. Forgive. That is the fourth rule to practice in learning to love.

Forgiving is not just an act of benevolence. It is a process, a procedure of freeing one's mind of resentment, bitterness, vengeance, and ill-will toward another.

Forgiving is such a vital component of mental health it has developed into a refined system of therapy in itself. To fully forgive may take a short time, or, in some cases, years. Professional help, counseling, support groups, or the love and interest of another may be needed. But, regardless of the depth and length of time, the process will remain essentially the same.

STEPS TO FORGIVE

This begins with the decision to forgive. The malice and pain have been endured long enough. There is an awareness that there can be no healing, no freedom, no serenity, no love without forgiveness.

There are reasons why it is seemingly impossible to decide to forgive.

The hurt, the resentment, the bitterness are so deeply entrenched they seem beyond healing by forgiveness.

It is sometimes assumed that to forgive would be to condone or endorse the merciless behavior of another.

Blaming others for setbacks and bruised feelings seems far more satisfying than forgiving.

Some acts are so despicable that they are thought to be "absolutely unforgivable."

A tendency always exists for people to make themselves right by making others wrong.

A sense of righteousness claims that antipathy and indignation will inflict punishment that another deserves. The offender is sentenced to permanent alienation by the words, "I will never, ever, forgive you for what you did."

Then, too, forgiving means giving up self-pity and the attention and sympathy it attracts.

So forgiveness is withheld and with it comes the pangs of self-inflicted malevolence. To lack forgiveness is to give another the power to cause pain and despair.

To live with the "piece of string" will have the same effect on one's life that it did on our French peasant, Master Hauchecorne. "He began to feel angry, worrying himself into a fever of irritation...but went on eating his heart out. Before the very eyes of people, he wasted away."

Choose to forgive. That starts the process of forgiving. No sacrifice is required. It won't hurt. And it could very well be the decision that puts your heart on the pathway to healing and enlightenment.

Choose to forgive. Then say it. "I forgive you." Aloud or silently. Indeed, silently may be best at times. For to say the words to another might only enflame old feelings. "Forgive me? Forgive me for what? It was all your fault."

Say them often to yourself. "I forgive you." Then, "I forgive myself. I forgive myself for my thoughts of vengeance, hostility, and resentment." These are cleansing statements. Repeat them often. They will nurture a tender mindfulness.

Turn the other cheek. For centuries this has symbolized the act of forgiving. In modern therapeutic language it would be termed a "shift in perspective." Substitute bad with good.

In the Adventures In Attitudes program, an exercise enables the participants to experience this perspective shift. They are asked to write down the name of a person who has treated them badly, for whom they might be carrying a grudge or resentment. Then they are told to write down as many good things as they can about the name written. A contest is held, the winner being the one who has the longest list of positive qualities.

That's part of the process of forgiving. Purge condemnation, criticism, and judgment.

Of similar nature I gave members of my classes in attitudes one of their more difficult assignments. "Next week," I told them, "help the person you dislike the most. Come back to our next meeting and tell us what happened."

The results were incredibly heart-warming. Typical was Harold, who had been having a two-year rift with his previous business partner. It had gone beyond a hot-tempered discord. They had suits pending in court against each other.

Harold came to class enthused and smiling. In response to the assignment of helping another, he reluctantly referred some business to the ex-partner. That was followed by a phone call of explanation. They talked. A date was set to have lunch together. At lunch, stubbornness melted. Argumentative issues were set aside. Friendship was restored. Both agreed to drop the lawsuits. They were healed.

You might consider the same assignment. Help the person you dislike the most.

Forgive. You have suffered enough. No longer need you give another the power to hurt you. You bring back your humanness and goodness by forgiving. It may be difficult. Perhaps you were treated badly. Keep in mind, though, that the injustice done to you could not possibly have been as severe as the brutality that wrenched out the words from the cross: "Forgive them, Father, for they know not what they do."

Think love. Speak love. Act love. Forgive. Four guidelines to follow to practice unconditional love.

TEACH LOVE

There is one more. Teach love. Why, oh why, must we be reminded of that? It should not be unfamiliar. Two thousand years ago, an itinerant preacher walked the shores of Galilee giving birth to unsurpassed ideas and new thoughts.

He spoke of the oneness of all. What you do to another is essentially done to yourself. Judge not for that is the manner in which you shall be judged.

The measurement of your concern for others shall be the measurement of their concern for you. Why look for the weaknesses in another without considering the faults within you? Set these aside first to see clearly how you can help another.

A new thought came forth for dealing with those who are against you. Love them. A person can be an enemy only when perceived as an enemy. If hate is replaced with love, if curses are substituted by blessings, if harm is dismissed by help, who, then, can be an enemy?

In a time when children and women were economic pawns and held in little honor it was a compassionate idea that all should be set free from suffering, servility and obscurity regardless of age, sex, or status.

It was a glorious revelation that the ill and deranged could be lifted from their illusions of sickness. This was not the touch of the miracle, but the natural ways of the soul's habitat. So was born fresh hope! The blind could see, the lame could walk, and the diseased could be healed!

There were new views expressed that were beyond the realities of the minds to which they were exposed. The seeing saw not; the hearing heard not; neither did they understand. Even in modern times, these principles are puzzling to many, beyond the grasp of what they believe.

So it was strange to hear that the kingdom of heaven was within. Heaven was described as being lovely, joyful, filled with wonder and love limited only by the dimension of human consciousness. It was explained that one need only accept this conviction and it would be as a seed growing into a tree of perfect life.

Hold in thought the kingdom of beauty, principle, love, righteousness, abundance and these shall be given to you. Dismiss the concerns of tomorrow for tomorrow shall be even more wondrous than today!

So the human being was declared to be empowered by love. The works that were seen done by one could be done in even greater proportion by all. That gave substance to the most omnipotent of the magnificent reflections—that the human being is, after all, a dream made in the image of the Creator of all ideas.

And it was good news that these majestic concepts were not born only in shrines, palaces, and hallowed walls, but came forth just as readily on grassy slopes and seashore pathways to those with open minds and hearts.

Think love. Speak love. Act love. Forgive. Teach love.

Love is eternal, lasting, the energy of life. Love shines. It is a beacon for life. That which contradicts love has no substance, nothing to support its existence. It fades in the light of love. Loving is getting in touch with your spirituality.

Strike out against discrimination, prejudice, and injustice in whatever form it takes. You don't need to join a crusade; just start with your own mind. When that gets clear, you can go on from there.

Of one thing you can be certain if you practice unconditional love. You will be empowered. You will be endowed with an embracing energy as real as the wind, the sun, and life itself.

That is why the fourth assignment for personal empowerment is, perhaps, one of the most important. Love unconditionally.

⟨⟩ Personal Empowerment ⟨⟩

Assignment Number Five

*"To The Degree You Give Others What They Need,
They Give You What You Need."*

TEN

People Need People

WE, THE NAMED AND UNNAMED, ARE THE PEOPLE OF YOUR LIFE.
We are the mirrors by which you know yourself.

Come, laugh with us when we laugh and cry with us when
we cry. Share our joys, our sorrows, our pleasures, and our pains. It
is your heart opening up to us that enriches your soul.

Like the acorn needing the soil, the moisture, and the air to
become an oak tree, you need us for your spirit to fulfill its destiny.

We, the people, give your life meaning and purpose. We add
value to your efforts and integrity to your character. Our very presence enables you to grow; we nurture and inspire you to do more
than you thought possible.

It is our love for you, spoken and unspoken, that heals, nourishes, and sustains your being. It is your love for us that glorifies your
mind, enhances your wholeness, and freshens your soul; without us
your divinity would stagnate like a pool of water that has no outlet.

We are your community—the music of your life. Alone we
are faintly heard; together we can be a symphony.

What is the meaning, the significance of community? Let's
look back through the windows of time and see one of the lionized
paradigms of community.

It is the 1800s. You are taking a short walk from the village
circle in Concord, Massachusetts. There reigns a majestic old colo-

nial home that was a spawning tributary for the world's philosophy and literature. Here, near the east coast of the United States, lived Ralph Waldo Emerson.

It was a home whose doors were always open to friends and neighbors wanting a bit of hospitality and conversation for a few hours or days. Henry David Thoreau, schoolteacher and writer, lived there for two years before returning to a hut beside Walden Pond, just a hike down the road from Emerson.

A few blocks in the other direction settled A. Bronson Alcott, vagrant peddler-turned-teacher who had been sacked from every teaching job he had held. His theories of education, far ahead of the times, may have been obscured forever by family poverty if not for the success of his daughter, Louisa May. Her writing, world-famed by *Little Women*, enabled Bronson to erect his own school and write a book titled, simply, *Ralph Waldo Emerson*.

Practically next door, secluded in a lofted room, Nathaniel Hawthorne was authoring such masterful works as *The Scarlet Letter* and *The House of Seven Gables*. Said to be the inspiration for his character, Zenobia, in *Blithedale Romance*, was another member of this select group, Margaret Fuller. Her writings and reform activities brought her notoriety spanning two continents.

Drifting in and out of this clan were such notables of the age as George Ripley and William Channing, liberal clergyman, inventor, and intellectual leader. Ripley withdrew from the ministry to organize Brook Farm, an experiment in communal living. Leaving that, he then founded *Harper's Magazine* and co-authored a set of encyclopedias.

Erase the eminent reputations these people achieved in history and it must be admitted that here was the elite "hippie" cult of its time. These were the reformers, the dissidents, the heady people reaching far out from the conventional.

One, Vern Jones, was even persuaded to enter an insane asylum, where he might have remained had it not been for Emerson, under whose patronage Jones went on to compose some of the most brilliant essays and poems of the period.

To stroll into the homes and habitat of these renowned in Concord is to recapture the pulse of that time and realize the enormous impact they had on each other. Apart from their literary and philosophical legacies, that might be the most valuable lesson bestowed to modern time.

They made each other better.

Each went different directions, but they urged one another to greatness in those paths. Through their moments together they nurtured, stimulated, and encouraged.

That was community at its best.

Nurturing Community

The results are as certain today as they were then. You are actualized by the people with whom you surround yourself. There are those who bring out your weaknesses. Better that the imperfections be unmasked to you than remain hidden. Then there are the cherished ones in whose presence you seem to be something better than you thought you could be. They nourish, excite, and enthuse you. These are the people who help you find the miracles that exist within you.

Find those people you can trust, who give you confidence, ones, perhaps, who aspire and exceed at being what you want to be. Or become bonded to others by a common purpose. Grow together. Let them stir you past horizons you never before reached.

That's community.

Who knows? You may sow seeds as significant as those in Concord in the 1800s. Not as far-reaching or celebrated, perhaps, but just as significant.

I was walking along the beach this morning in Hawaii thinking about community. There were groups of sandpipers flicking back and forth on their spindly legs. Out at sea were some humpbacks lazily rolling along, occasionally breaking water. Overhead, a formation of gulls was riding the billows of the trade winds.

All about me was life. But it was together; the birds were in flocks; the whales were a pod. That seems to be an inherent characteristic of life, a tendency toward community. When the group disintegrates, falls apart, each isolated from the other, that form of life gradually dies, becomes extinct.

Does that same need rest in the crevices of the human being? Is there a deep abiding hunger for community, being together, a bonding one for another? When denied, does that same tendency toward extinction cannibalize us? Does a part of us begin to erode?

Is that what is happening in our society? Are there no commitments as people drift from one relationship to another? Do separate careers keep couples apart, parents pulled out of the home by work? Is prosperity leading people to look for thrills and amusement outside rather than in the home? Are these some of the unseen forces wrenching our society, causing a deterioration of community? I ask the questions; I'm not sure I know the answers.

When Nadine and I were first married we bought an old house with a small down payment. Carpeting, washer, dryer, and a car were purchased with monthly payments. Soon, there were a couple more mouths. There never seemed to be much money left at the end of the month; indeed, there was always a lot of month left at the end of the money.

But we were not alone. All those about us were experiencing the same state of affairs. So we became community. We ate together, played games together, celebrated holidays in the back yards, tended each others' children, and supported each other in our setbacks and sorrows. Treasured memories and friendships were rooted that have endured for years.

That was community. It was also one of my classrooms in the school of life. The subject was "the influence of people on our lives." That class, coupled with a budding career involving people, made me realize the incredible effect people have on one another.

THE POWER OF THE PEOPLE

People need people. People empower people. But to be empowered by people, first empower them. Therein lies the fifth assignment for personal empowerment: "To the degree you give others what they need, they will give you what you need."

I did not originate the principle. It surfaced after a two-day seminar I was conducting at the University of Wisconsin. It was staged for management personnel; subjects included attitude assessment, motivation, persuasion, and supervision.

Bill Stilwell, representing the University, was auditing the program. In a few brief remarks to close out the session Bill said, "It seems to me that everything that has been said here in the last two days can be summed up in just one sentence. 'To the degree you give others what they need, they will give you what you need!'"

What an insight! I wish I had said it. But that doesn't mean I can't own it. I have. And so can you. You will discover, as I have, that it is the key to persuading, motivating, leading, supervising, influencing, parenting, and building meaningful relationships and community.

Give people what they need. Do that first. That's important. George will tell you that. Good neighbor George, you see, was the parking lot for his friends' troubles. He had an attentive ear and usually some comforting advice.

A pal was laying his sad story on George one day. "I can't live with that wife of mine another moment. She's cold, silent, critical, or nagging all the time. I'm leaving her as soon as I can. I'll give her a dose of the misery she's been giving me!"

George said, "You're not going to do that if you leave her while you're mad. She'll be glad to be rid of you. If you want to shake her up, stop on the way home for some flowers and candy. Walk in the front door smiling. Tell her how attractive she is. Be loving, kind, gentle, regardless of what she does to you. Make yourself indispensable for the next 30 days. Then leave her. That'll really hurt her."

A month later George met the friend again who blurted out, "How come you didn't tell me you talked to my wife? I did just what you told me to do. I know you talked to her because she started treating me the same way I acted towards her. Now I couldn't live without her."

You've got it right, George. Fill others' needs first; then they fill yours. There's a multitude of lonely people out there who are trying to work the rule backwards. They're saying, "Meet my needs first, then I'll think about yours." They're coming up empty.

There is an ancient Persian proverb that expresses the idea more specifically: "If you seek a brother to share your burden, brothers are in truth hard to find. But if you are in search of some-

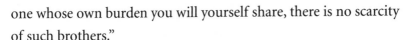

one whose own burden you will yourself share, there is no scarcity of such brothers."

Notice, too, that the rule states: "To the degree you give others what they need..." Need, not want.

Wants and needs are separate substances. Wants are frivolous, itchy, plundering, often greedy forces that are never satisfied. Meet one want, and there are two more to replace it.

But needs are the deeper currents of one's existence. They are meaningful, worthy, and not as capricious as wants.

People want sympathy; they need empathy.

People want riches; they need fulfillment.

People want big cars and expensive homes; they need transportation and shelter.

People want fame; they need recognition.

People want power; they need support and cooperation.

People want to dominate; they need to influence and guide.

People want prestige, they need respect.

Children want freedom and permissiveness; they need discipline.

People want ease and comfort; they need achievement and work.

People want adoration; they need love.

So, "To the degree you give others what they need, they will give you what you need."

What do others need? Look well within yourself, and you will find that which exists in others. What you need, they need. What is closest to your heart, emotionally, is also closest to theirs. You are your own barometer, your own measuring device, of what you need to give in order to get what you need from life.

In his *Essay on Self-Reliance*, Ralph Waldo Emerson wrote,

"To believe your own thought, to believe that what is true for you in your private heart is true for all people—that is genius."

DEFINE YOUR NEEDS

What is it stirring about in your mind and heart that reaches out for another? First is a yearning for someone, as you wander through life, who cares about you—someone who picks you out of the crowd, notices you, remembers you, makes you feel you're someone special. This is a person whose companionship you enjoy, one with whom you can share your triumphs and gladness. One, also, who will be there to help bear your sadness or troubles.

We're describing a friend, aren't we? You need a friend, a person you can trust, one with whom you can lift the veil of privacy, relax, and be yourself without risk, judgment, or criticism. With a friend there is no criticism. With a friend there is no need to tiptoe around on eggshells trying to say the right things and carefully avoiding the wrong things.

Between friends there is no competition. Left behind is a comparison of whose children are brightest or most lovable, whose home is the largest, or whose car is most expensive. Friends don't compete; they find joy in each others' successes and sorrow in the others' defeat.

A friend is one who listens. That, above all else, is the symbol of friendship. Listening. It is also an empowering strategy. For you have a greater effect on people by the way that you listen than the way that you talk. Most people don't realize that. They believe that they are empowered by the way they talk and have little concern about their listening ability.

This became apparent some years ago when I was involved with a course in public speaking in the adult education program of the Minneapolis public schools. The subject became so popular that we had to recruit two additional teachers to handle the people who registered.

Concurrent with these programs, over a four-year period, a listening course was offered. It was never conducted. Only a half dozen or so indicated any interest in it, never enough to make up a class!

Everyone wanted to learn how to talk! No one wanted to learn how to listen! Only a sparse half dozen had any inkling that listening presented any difficulty—that it is a critical link in interpersonal relationships.

From a flat on Vienna's Bergasse many years ago came testimony that talking about oneself and having another listen is not only comforting but, at times, almost lifesaving.

Herr Doktor Freud discovered that merely talking about one's inner emotions and the tangle of life's experiences can be healing therapy. Freud's therapeutic technique of psychoanalysis, letting the patient talk, opened a new era of psychology. Today, of course, it is the base for all counseling and psychological treatment of any sort.

How do you become a better listener? It's so self-evident that there is an inclination to assume that it's easy.

You must *want* to listen.

You must lather up a keen desire to hear what the other person has to say.

Lukewarm listeners don't have an intellectual problem; they have an emotional problem. They lack the mental appetite for listening, being so preoccupied with themselves that others' words are completely tuned out.

But that's an emotional hang-up. It's not because they don't know how to listen. They just don't want to.

If you were compelled to take a course in parachute packing, you'd probably find it quite dull. Your attention would wander.

But if you were told that tomorrow you would be forced to pack your own chute and jump from an airplane, your earlobes would virtually vibrate with the strain of listening. Your life would dangle on being able to catch every word of the instructor.

Maybe staying alive won't depend on your listening skills, but your ability to be a friend, giving others what they need, certainly does.

TOUGH LISTENING

If you see yourself as one who likes to listen, you might be thinking of social situations, the give-and-take chitchat that occurs when interesting little tidbits are being exchanged. But there are times when fears, prejudices, anxieties, preoccupation, self-concern, and the unbridled compulsion to talk all stand as roadblocks to productive listening. To set these aside is difficult; it's tough listening.

Tough listening is when one of your kids starts running down your value concepts, picking away at some of the standards that you feel are so vital to being a contributing member of the human race. You're inclined to blast away. The only thing holding you back is the realization that you'll be slamming the door on any future open communication. But it's tough listening.

Tough listening is letting a friend rip apart your glimmering political hero. You've got all the facts and figures to prove how wrong the friend is. But reciting your opinion isn't going to enrich the friendship. Listening is. Tough listening, that is.

Tough listening is getting the shaggy stuff out in the air in a love relationship. You're being judged and accused of some guff that you regard as unfair or untrue. You hurt. The first inclination is to hurt back. But that isn't going to help the other person be your friend. Tough listening will.

Tough listening is sitting in on the church's building improvement committee as they discuss taking out the dahlia bed and honeysuckle hedge and putting in a parking lot. You're violently opposed and are squirming with fifteen aesthetic, financial, and logical reasons why it should not be done. But lashing out at the other members, cutting their rationale to bits, won't put them in your camp. Studied listening and patient reasoning will. But it's tough listening.

Tough listening is putting the clamps on that compelling anxiety to express yourself. It's a strain on self-discipline at times. Indeed, simply restraining your verbal velocity isn't enough. Rise higher to demonstrate the qualities of intent, active listening.

I don't have to tell you how to do that. You know. Look around you. Notice the traits of the people with whom you enjoy visiting, the good listeners.

They show their interest with their eyes, posture, and the ways that they react. At times they might smile, raise the eyebrows, and nod their heads in agreement. It's a sort of indescribable mood that says, "I enjoy listening to you. You're important to me."

Don't come to the conclusion that effective listening is being perched like a sphinx while another rambles on. Nothing would be more boring than two people doing that to each other.

Listening should not inhibit self-expression, give-and-take, mixing and watching, feeling and talking, the depth and joy of people using the gift of verbalizing to share their experiences and opinions. Situations and people vary. You have to get a handle on when you should talk and when you should listen.

Just be concerned about the other person's needs and interests. When a person can be relaxed in your presence, letting out whatever is inside, pausing, thinking, skipping, starting over, stammering a little, going back and forth spurred on by the glow of interest in your eyes—that's great listening!

Do that and you will never lack for a friend. It's another way of versing the old adage: "To have a friend, be one."

BEING A FRIEND

Waiting hungrily, perhaps silently, are a host of people longing for your friendship. Long ago they were girls or boys like Tommy. The kids called Tommy "fatty." The teachers told him he was lazy, capable of better work. His mother nagged him about his sloppy appearance. He didn't go to school dances; he knew no one would want to dance with him. Besides, the girls would just make fun of him. He got laughed at in gym class because he was awkward and slow. Tommy wanted to study art; his dad bugged him to take business courses.

Tommy struggled through all the rejection, criticism, blemishes on the face, braces on the teeth, and grew up.

Now you come along. You look past the shyness, the pounds on the hips, the spectacles, and the misshapen nose. You become a lot of people to Tommy—the people he wanted to impress but couldn't. You talk about his warm smile, artistic talents, secret ambitions, and keen sensitivity to others.

You suddenly become for Tommy a parent who had time to listen, a teacher who talked about what was right about him instead of pointing out mistakes, a coach who put him in the game instead of keeping him on the sidelines, and, above all, a friend who was interested in him rather than what he looked like.

That attitude, in itself, can have a profound effect on others. Just look at them as capable, feeling, worthwhile human beings.

The story is told of the banker who often dropped a coin in the cup of the legless beggar who sat on the street outside the bank. But, unlike most people, the banker would always insist on getting one of the pencils the pauper had beside him. "You are a merchant," the banker would say, "and I always expect to receive good value from merchants I do business with."

One day the squat, hunched figure was not on the sidewalk. Time passed and the banker forgot about him, until he walked into a public building and there in the concessions stand sat the former vagrant. "I have always hoped you might come by someday," the storekeeper remarked. "You are largely responsible for me being here. You kept telling me I was a 'merchant.' I started thinking of myself that way, instead of a beggar receiving gifts. I started selling pencils—lots of them. You gave me self-respect, caused me to look at myself differently."

How do you see others? Do you view them critically, letting yourself be disturbed with the defects, failings, and traits they lack? Or do you see the goodness and wonders of people?

Do you perceive the beggar or the merchant in those about you?

Behind the masks that others wear from day to day is a little of the beggar or the Tommy. No matter how rich, famous, or successful they might appear, there is a hollowness that longs to be filled. Put a bit of you in that emptiness and the passing faces start pausing to look toward you. Those who have been far away are suddenly close. The world becomes a friendly place that meets your every need and wish before they are even expressed. People respond favorably; they become your community. You empower them; they empower you.

The Importance of Appreciation

What else do people need that you can give them?

Although the nation has done a fair job of feeding the populace physically, there are millions going to bed every night starving emotionally for a few words or gestures of appreciation.

At the time the famed psychologist William James was working on his book, he was taken ill and confined to the hospital. A friend sent him an azalea plant and a note of appreciation. In expressing thanks for the plant, Dr. James said it brought to his attention an omission from his book.

He said he had neglected *the deepest quality of human nature—the craving to be appreciated!*

Giving appreciation makes the other person feel wanted, loved, needed. It helps one to like oneself.

Studies have shown that there is more job dissatisfaction caused by lack of appreciation than all other causes combined!

Surveys indicate that the greatest factor in marital tension is the inability of a partner to show appreciation.

The story is told of the woman who had worked hard raising a family with little appreciation from the family.

One evening she asked her husband, "I suppose, Peter, that if I should die you would spend a large amount for flowers for me, wouldn't you?"

"Of course I would, Martha. Why do you ask?"

"I was just thinking that the wreaths would mean very little to me then. But just one little flower from time to time while I am living would mean so much to me."

Wasn't Martha really voicing the heartfelt hunger throbbing within the breast of all the people you see? "Just a little flower from time to time" gives people the basic hope and joy of their living.

Why wait until the hearts have stopped loving, the eyes are unseeing, and the ears are not listening?

A gifted executive, looking back on his career, realized how greatly his life had been influenced as a youth by a certain teacher. He traced her through the school, found that she was retired, and wrote her of his appreciation.

He received this reply:

"I can't tell you how much your note meant to me. I am in my eighties, living alone in a small room, cooking my own meals, lonely, and like the last leaf of fall lingering behind. You will be interested to know that I taught school for fifty years and yours is the first note of appreciation I have ever received. It came to me on a blue, cold morning, and it cheered me as nothing has in years."

"It cheered me as nothing has in years!" That sentence is a jolting revelation of the longing that people have for appreciation.

Are you generous with your appreciation for others? You are the child of all whom you have known. Each has woven in a bit of the color that makes the pattern of who you are. Search beyond the shallowness of false pride and, like the executive who wrote the schoolteacher, recognize the contributions others have made to your existence.

Cherish those who have touched your life and, in so doing, pressed you into being what you are today. They, in their stumbling, fumbling ways may have caused you to cry or rebel or fret with anger. Their love and concern might have been disguised with impatience, criticism, restriction, and worry. But those are only indications that they cared. So gaze about you. Who can you find to appreciate?

BE GENEROUS WITH PRAISE

People crave appreciation. But is that enough? No. Their

needs go beyond that. They want to stand out, be noticed, made to feel important. Recognition, a few ribbons tagged on their chests, does that for them.

The efforts to get special attention start at an early age. "Come here, Mommy. Look at the sand castle I made," cries the child at the beach.

The tiny face peeking around the corner of the newspaper, a tug on the pants leg, the beaming smile of pride that goes with the freshly picked bouquet of dandelions are all simple requests saying, "Notice me!"

A substantial part of children's behavior that parents might call "naughtiness" is only the outcropping of the wish for recognition. It doesn't end when school starts. the results of giving recognition to children in the classroom are so overwhelmingly positive that it is accepted as the significant stimulant to learning.

Gold stars, being the class messenger to the principal's office, special privileges, a name on a blackboard, a compliment, and all the many other ways of recognizing children, making them feel important, are part of the spawning process in which those little humans flourish.

A psychologist once told me, "There is no mystery to raising children. Just praise them. When they eat right, praise them. When they draw a picture, praise them. When they learn to ride a bike, praise them."

Denying attention to children is rejection. That creates antagonism, anti-social attitudes, all sorts of behavior problems. Nothing very complicated about it. Rejection is painful. Recognition pleases, heals.

It's a characteristic that never changes much in the life cycle. Phillip Brooks said it this way: "To say, 'well done' to any bit of good work is to take hold of the powers which have made the effort and strengthen them beyond our knowledge!"

"We are all excited by the love of praise," wrote Cicero.

Praise spurs people to achieve, gives them inner confidence, and makes them grow.

There are dozens of ways to recognize people, to put them on a pedestal and stroke the egos that the world so customarily ignores. It is of vital significance that you emphasize the uniqueness and wonder of every human being you meet. You will never fully comprehend the impact you can have on others' lives by building them up by special recognition.

Give thoughtful attention to every person's matchless qualities, not just certain people with whom you want to ingratiate yourself.

All people are beautiful and special. Practice making them feel that way.

The waitress who serves you a cup of coffee, the elevator operator, the clerk, the boss, the next-door neighbor, the stranger you pass on the street, the man who comes to pick up your garbage, the janitor who cares for your office building, the child who delivers your paper, the teacher, the preacher, the barber, the mail carrier— the whole panorama of people who enter your life for only brief moments—all are worth the thoughtful effort it takes to make them feel important!

Incidentally, be prepared to feel pretty good about yourself. Because what you give to others is going to be given back to you!

YOU ARE RIGHT

Consider one other need that people have. They need to be right. Lurking in the human psyche is a malicious little voice that is constantly compelling us to prove that we are right and the world or the other person is wrong. It has probably destroyed more relationships and distorted more lives than any other trait.

It is a tendency that has been hanging around in the crevices of humanity since the dinosaur days. The human being has very few natural defenses as compared with other forms of life. Our prehistoric ancestors did not have the strength of bears, the venom of snakes, the needles of porcupines, the fangs of wolves, or, hopefully, the odors of skunks. The only defense of the human was the mind. The very existence of life was dependent on making the right decisions when faced with danger or life-threatening situations; the human mind responded by believing it had to be right to survive. It has not changed much. Deeply imbedded in the thought process is the conviction that to survive one must be right. To preserve that dogma in interpersonal relationships requires that the other person be wrong. In fact, that urge becomes so strong at times that it overshadows all aspects of the relationship.

Wars, pain, strife, energy, and assorted other distresses are wasted on the struggle to be right.

Observe, for instance, the sickness that plagues our freeways. Shootings, horn honking, obscene gestures, and physical violence occur as ways of telling another driver, "You're driving wrong."

There has never been a soul who, at some time, has not felt under-appreciated and overworked. To allow that feeling to grow is to go to some strong extremes to prove that others are wrong. Alas! How many careers are detoured and marriage relationships aborted by the tenacious struggle to be right?

The futility of hanging on to the "I'm right! You're wrong!" syndrome almost always prevails. It is rarely achieved in relationships. Think, for a moment, about the last disagreement you had with someone. Who was right? You were, weren't you? And the more you thought about it the more right you became. And, odds are, the other person was hanging on to the same conviction of being right.

Here's a simple suggestion for turning this bias around and making it work for you rather than against you. Help the other person be right! When confronted by a situation in which you are tempted to attack another's view, say to yourself, "I'm wrong. You're right." You don't have to hang onto it forever. Just hold it in your mind long enough to see the other person's perspective.

If there is a difference of opinion with another, don't fall into the "I'm right. You're wrong" trap. Instead, work towards determining *what* is right, rather than *who* is right. In fact, those are velvet-like words to open negotiations. Try suggesting, "It's not important to prove who is right or who is wrong. What we want to decide is what is right and go from there."

People are rarely totally wrong or totally right. Find the ways that others are right and stress those points. You will find them much less adamant about defending their differences with you.

Avoid sentences that imply that you are going to get into an "I'm right. You're wrong." stance. Here are a few of those:

"You should have…"

"I knew this would happen."

"Why didn't you…?"

"You neglected to…"

"If you had mentioned that before…"

"This never would have happened if you had…"

"You were supposed to…"

Remember that in almost all instances of differences of opinion you are not dealing with facts. You are dealing with attitudes and views. Shakespeare reminded us of that when he wrote: *"There is nothing right or wrong, but thinking makes it so."*

It Is Up to You

People are always reacting to you—negatively, positively, or passively. Those reactions are somewhat dependent on your appearance and personality, but most reactions of a deeper nature are influenced by your attitudes and actions towards others. That responsibility may be likened to the fable that is told of the elderly mystic who had perfect knowledge and insight of all things. When asked a question, he had never been known to give a wrong answer.

One day one of the boys in the village gathered the other boys about him. "I have at last thought of a question," he boasted, "that the ancient Wise One will be unable to answer correctly.

"I have captured a small bird. I shall go to the Wise One with the bird concealed in my hands. I shall ask him if the bird is alive or dead. If he says the bird is alive I shall crush the bird in my hands and throw it, dead, at his feet. If he says the bird is dead, I shall open my hands and the bird shall fly away."

With that, the boys went forth to the place of the Wise One. On arrival the boy asked, "Tell me, O Wise One, is the bird that I have in my hands alive or dead?"

The elderly sage pondered a moment and then responded, "The answer, my son, rests in your hands!"

So it is with building relationships. The answer rests in your hands.

Nourishing friendships, community, and transactions with others that empower rests in your dedication to the fifth assignment—"To the degree you give others what they need, they will give you what you need."

That's really very simple isn't it? The more you give, the more empowered you become. It's remindful of the man in a desolate mountain region who was a laborer six days a week and a preacher on the seventh. He served a small rural congregation tucked far up in the hills. The only monetary compensation he got came from the morning offering. One Sunday, his six-year-old daughter went along with him to the service. Just inside the door of the small frame church was a table, and on it rested a collection basket. As they entered, the daughter saw her father place a half-dollar in the wicker basket before any of the people arrived.

When the service had ended and the last member had departed, the parson and his daughter started to leave. As they reached the door, both peered expectantly into the collection basket and found that the only "take" was the half-dollar he had donated.

After a short silence the little girl said, "You know, Daddy, if you had put more in, you'd have gotten more out!"

∽ PERSONAL EMPOWERMENT ∽

ASSIGNMENT NUMBER SIX

*"Visualize
Verbalize
Vitalize"*

ELEVEN

Capture the Vision

"THE ACTIVITIES OF THE MIND HAVE NO LIMIT, THEY FORM THE SURROUNDINGS OF LIFE. An impure mind surrounds itself with impure things and a pure mind surrounds itself with pure things. Just as a picture is drawn by an artist, surroundings are created by the activities of the mind.

"Human beings tend to move in the directions of their thoughts. If they harbor greedy thoughts, they become more greedy; if they think angry thoughts, they become more angry; if they hold thoughts of revenge their feet move in that direction."

Those words are neither recent nor original. They are quotes from *The Teaching of Buddha*, written more than 2,500 years ago. The philosophy advises that to control the mind is to control life. A bewildered life rises out of a bewildered mind, a mind that is "never free from memories, fears, or laments, not only in the past but the present and future."

Such seeds, buried in the soils of one's consciousness, will grow into sickness, neuroses, and irrational behavior.

So what's new? Nothing, really. All of what is being discussed in seminars, management clinics, therapy sessions, personal growth programs, and psychological disciplines is little more than data that has been reworked out of ancient wisdom.

That, in itself, can be enormously enlightening. In the rustle and hustle to absorb the latest information about growing rich, dodging a divorce, shedding childhood phobias, gaining power over others, or career success, one gets mixed in waist-high complexities. Completely overlooked is the very simple concept of changing one's life by changing one's thoughts.

It has never been expressed more clearly than by James Allen in his memorable essay, "As A Man Thinketh." He wrote:

"As the plant springs from, and could not be without, the seed, so every act of a person springs from the hidden seeds of thought, and could not have appeared without them. Act is the blossom of thought, and joy and suffering are its fruits.

"A person's mind may be likened to a garden, which may be intelligently cultivated or allowed to run wild; but whether cultivated or neglected, it must, and will, bring forth. If no useful seeds are put into it, then an abundance of useless weed-seeds will fall therein, and will continue to produce their kind.

"Just as a gardener cultivates the plot, keeping it free from weeds, and growing flowers and fruits, so may a person tend the garden of mind, weeding out all the wrong, useless, and impure thoughts, and cultivating toward perfection the flowers and fruits of right, useful, and pure thoughts."

Wonderful! All we have to do to build a magnificent life is to generate positive thoughts and actions and they become reality.

It sounds simple; but it isn't always easy. Because thoughts are too often like feathers blown around in the mind by outside forces, many of which are frightfully destructive.

Our minds are like high-fidelity recorders. They record experiences, words, ideas, and events to which we are exposed. These are never erased. They play back and become reality. Many negative recordings are so deeply embedded we do not even recognize they exist.

Our lives as babies are our only thoroughly positive experiences. Then we are loved. Totally loved. When we start walking we are restrained, punished, criticized, disciplined, and molded by well-intentioned adults. In the youthful mind this often spawns defiance, resistance, and hostility. The love as it was once known is missing.

We grow up in a society based on materialistic values. Success is making money; happiness and security become financially oriented. So we find ourselves competing—not only for money, position, and power but also for recognition, acceptance, and love. In our culture, competition is encouraged. It becomes a virtue. So relationships can become contests. Someone wins, and someone loses. Or someone is charging us too much or paying us too little.

We are taught to beware of strangers. We lock ourselves inside our homes at night. As children we are told to strike back when struck. Our language is filled with *fight*—"fight for what is yours"; "fight for success." Toys are sometimes guns and lethal devices; games are "cops and robbers." Crime and violence become a source of sordid interest and pleasure. Newspapers, movies, and TV shows are filled with such diabolical stories.

Attitudes can become antagonistic, suspicious, belligerent, sometimes angry and hateful toward others.

The environment can become our enemy. It is polluted. It is filled with smog, drafts, smoke, pollens, and humidity that we are told are harmful. We hate bugs, weeds, germs, and dirt. We sterilize, sanitize, and fill the air, our yards, and our homes with toxic materials.

In our search for comfort we find days too hot or too cold, too wet or too dry. So we must control the temperature to control our mood.

TVs and newspapers warn us about heart attacks, cancer, headaches, stomach gas, and a variety of other ills and dangers.

We are overwhelmed with information about the things that make us sick; so we think more about sickness than about health.

Those are the perspectives from which attitudes are created. Strangely, the human mind clutches tenaciously to those paradigms as reality.

"But that's the way the world really is," a voice within proclaims. Yes. All negative thoughts are self-confirming. They can be justified. But they do not make life better. Mixed in with daily activities they subtract a big chunk of life's potentials.

Is there a solution? There is. Choose your attitudes. Control your thoughts. Learn to manage your mind. There is only one formula, one method for doing that. You can deaden or numb the mind or put it into contortions with pills or substances but there is only one process of mind-management. That involves three principles: "visualize, verbalize, vitalize." Those, then, become the sixth assignment.

Practicing those techniques will empower you to choose your thoughts and free yourself of the negativism that tries to invade your consciousness. As Victor Frankl proclaimed in his *Man's Search For Meaning*, "...your ultimate freedom is the ability to choose your attitudes in any given set of circumstances."

We call it the "3V" formula for managing the mind. Visualize! Verbalize! Vitalize!

Let's start with "visualize."

THE POWER OF VISUALIZATION

During attitude assessment seminars I asked participants to write down how they pictured themselves, suggesting that they begin with the words "I am." Out of hundreds of responses here are a few that are typical:

1. "Who am I? I am a slightly overweight, slightly lazy individual. I enjoy recreational activities more than constructive activities. I am happily married. I am somewhat scared about a number of things. I consider myself an average sort of fellow."

2. "I am quiet and unassuming. I am above average in intelligence. I would like to be liked but I am unable to communicate my personality to most other people. To most other people who I don't know very well I appear as a kind of neurotic. This is one fault I must overcome."

3. "I think I try to do more than expected. I am over-emotional and especially when I don't have a system or set of procedures and guides for what I'm supposed to do. I am somewhat insecure because I haven't had much experience. I don't know exactly what I have to do to keep my present job or what performance my superiors want. But I try."

4. "I work hard when I want something. Otherwise, I go along with the daily routines."

5. "I frankly don't think I can answer."

6. "I am a young man recently out of school, working in a full-time position. I have a rural background and relatively rural values."

7. "I am rather restless, but I have the determination to settle down. I am also a product of post-war Europe with attitudes sometimes differing from those I encounter here. Therefore, I'm continuously undoing my attitudes."

8. "A school teacher with most of my future behind me."

9. "I am a man who likes things mechanical. I don't like to get up early but like to go to bed late. I'm more or less talkative but not too interesting to most people. I think I'm a little mixed up."

10. "I think of me as just a person. I'm a beautician, twenty-nine years old, a woman, a human being."

11. "I think I'm hard working. But I'm unoriented to a good goal. I try to be dependable."

12. "I picture myself as a male of the human race. I'm a citizen. I have a job. I'm married."

All of these well-intentioned people, like so many others, might lift themselves from what Thoreau described as "lives of quiet desperation" by use of their imaginations—visualizing.

They could learn from a beautiful old story about a Persian prince born a hunchback. In all other ways the child was remarkable.

He had a sharp mind, was well-coordinated, and was ambitious beyond his years. He was endowed with a pride for his family position but sensitive of his physical limitation.

On his twelfth birthday his father said, "It is your twelfth birthday, son. It is an important one because you pass the portals of childhood. Tell me, what would you like most of all on your birthday?"

And the proud king was somewhat dismayed at his son's lack of humility when the boy answered that he would like a statue of himself.

The finest marble was obtained, and the king secured the services of the most skilled sculptor in the kingdom. But then the boy sought counsel with the sculptor. He demanded that the statue not be made as he actually was but, instead, carved with a perfect body, straight and well shaped.

The statue was finished as the prince directed. Then it was placed on a pedestal in the palace gardens.

At the beginning of each day and just before going to bed at night the prince stood before the statue and said, "This is me. This is the way I shall grow up. This is my face, my body. This is the way I shall look to others!"

A dream became a vision; a vision became a picture; and the picture became rooted deep in the prince's mind and heart. It was fused with desire and emotion. Each night he stretched out straighter in his bed. Each day he walked a bit more erect.

And, as he grew into manhood, he became exactly like the statue, straight and tall, perfect in body and stature!

The world is full of "Persian princes" who have discovered the molding impact of visualization—carrying in the mind the pictures of the persons they would like to be.

John F. Kennedy wanted to be President of the United States. His idol was Franklin Roosevelt.

As a young man, John Kennedy carried the picture of Franklin Roosevelt in his mind. He studied Roosevelt, his programs, his personality.

John Kennedy acted out the picture in his mind, became President of the United States, and instigated programs resembling those of Roosevelt.

A noted plastic surgeon, Dr. Maxwell Maltz, discovered that the human mind is like a computer in many respects. The mind returns the pictures it is fed. He describes the principles of visualization in his book *Psycho-Cybernetics*. In it he says:

"Each of us has a mental picture of himself, a self-image which governs much of his conduct and outlook. To find life reasonably satisfying you must have a self-image that you can life with. You must find yourself acceptable to you. You must have a self that you like, and one that you can trust and believe in.

"When this self-image is one you can be proud of, you feel self-confident. You feel free to be yourself and to express yourself. You function at your best. When the self-image is an object of shame, you attempt to hide it rather than express it. Creative expression is blocked. You become hostile and hard to get along with.

"As a plastic surgeon, I used to be amazed by the dramatic and sudden changes in character and personality which often resulted when a facial defect (usually crucial to the patient's self-image) had been corrected. Sometimes the operation appeared to create an entirely new person, transforming not only the patient's appearance but also his whole life.

"The shy and retiring, once rid of their disfigurement, became bold and courageous. A 'moronic' boy changed into an alert, bright and ambitious youngster when I corrected the too-large ears that had invited chronic ridicule. A salesman, obsessed by the conviction that he was repulsive to others because an automobile accident had left him horribly scarred, became a model of self-confidence when the scars were removed. Most startling of all, an incorrigible habitual criminal lost his bitter defiance almost overnight, won a parole and went on to assume a responsible role in society."

Studies done some time ago by Professor K. P. Koenig at Stanford University indicate the strength mental pictures have in human behavior.

He used three study groups to examine techniques for breaking the habit of cigarette smoking.

On the first group he used the "Freudian" method of psychological counseling. The group discussed, analyzed, and attempted to gain insight into their acquired habit of smoking.

About 50 percent of them gave up smoking as a result.

On the second group, Dr. Koenig used the "conditioned response" method. At unpredictable times when they were smoking they would receive an electric shock. It was expected that they would begin to associate smoking with fear, shock, and general unpleasantness. One disadvantage was that the students didn't like it; they dropped out of the experiment. But it was 63 percent effective in accomplishing a reduction in smoking in the remaining group.

But a new technique was tried on the third group. They were told to develop mental pictures of their favorite smoking situations. They visualized themselves drinking coffee, just completing breakfast, having a break in the student grill, or any of their other favorite smoke times.

But they were asked to picture themselves enjoying these situations *without a cigarette!* They were trained to imagine themselves, essentially, enjoying *not* smoking.

This group showed a *75 percent reduction in smoking!*

Visualization proved to be the most effective influence over their behavior habit!

A lady in one of my "Adventures In Attitudes" put to work the concept of visualization with her son who was failing in junior high school.

She got a blank report card from the principal. And filled it with As and Bs. She put the card up in the boy's room. Beside the card she hung a picture of the boy behind a desk with a textbook. She then helped her son develop a picture of himself as a top student, handing in fine work, and getting good grades on tests.

The boy's work showed sharp improvement. Every test that was an A or B was mounted on the wall in the boy's room.

Six weeks later he received a report card with only one grade on it lower than an A or a B!

This may not work for everyone but it's worth considering, isn't it?

MENTAL PICTURES BECOME REALITY

There can be no more significant revelation for personal empowerment than this: Your subliminal self, the driving force of your life, thinks in imagery with an incredible impact on behavior.

Television has become such a powerful advertising force because of the image it is able to project on your mind. You are put into a convertible car for a carefree drive along scenic, winding roadways by an auto manufacturer. The airlines can carry you through friendly skies to fascinating treks in the Far East. Or you are a smiling nymph of a woman frolicking through a day's housework if you use the soap suggested on your screen.

The full power of these pictures in your subconscious come into focus when you buy. You find yourself fulfilling the picture in your subconscious by purchasing the products suggested without *consciously* realizing why you are buying.

The effect of the consumer's subconscious mind on the buying act has opened a vast new area of research, sometimes described as "depth motivation" or the "depth approach." These simply recognize that your actions are not always logical, rational, and carefully deliberated at the conscious level; *there is an impulsive effort for one to act out the pictures hung in the subconscious mind!*

It is amazing that the power of the subconscious picture in

human behavior and attitude was not brought into full focus before! The Bible refers to mental "visions" 102 different times; Confucius said, "One picture is worth 10,000 words"; and Aesop's simple fables of moral behavior delineated pictures that have hung in the subconscious minds of millions from childhood to old age.

All "memory systems" depend on the power and permanency of mental pictures. Most people try to "memorize," using their conscious minds, and rebel at the realization that they have a "bad memory." The experts make no attempt to "memorize" at all; they simply hang a mental picture and recall it when they want it. Their genius lies in their ability to develop the mental image systems for numbers, name sequences, and words.

Visualization is attracting ever-growing attention as a healing mechanism for mental and physical disorders. It has become almost standard therapy for cancer patients resulting in many remarkable instances of remission.

Dr. O. Carl Simonton, the forerunner of these procedures, supplements standard medical practices with visual imagery for treatment of cancer. He instructs those afflicted to visualize the body's immune mechanism combating the disease.

"Think of the cancer cells," he advises, "as something soft that can be broken down like hamburger meat."

Ralph, a participant in my attitude development group, shared a personal experience with me one evening after the class.

"I was formerly a clerk with a small company in this city. I spent eight years in exactly the same job. I had four small raises in that time. I often felt I should quit my job and look for something better. But I didn't have enough confidence in myself to think any other company wanted me.

"And then the roof fell in!" Ralph continued. "This small

company was bought out. They broke the news that many of us would have to go. I was told I was one of them!

"I became desperate and I did a rather foolish thing. I went to the company head. I pleaded with him to give me some kind of job. This was the only work I knew. I told him I would work at anything for any amount of money.

"He said he would pass the word along. Well, he did. And they reconsidered. They hired me back to do twice the work at *half the pay.*"

Ralph shook his head as he recalled the unpleasant memories. "I was mad at myself," he remarked. "The shame of going through that just to hang on to work got to me. It would have been different if we were in the depths of depression. But we weren't. This was prosperity. Others were enjoying the plenty of a thriving nation.

"I was really ready for what was to happen to me. A friend loaned me a copy of a book he had. In the book was written the importance of how we think of ourselves—the image of who we are. It pointed out that most of us have feelings of inferiority. We pick out our faults to paint our mental self-portrait. Then we simply project these into the future.

"That hit the nail on the head with me!" exclaimed Ralph. "But this book told how a person could change his self-image and as a result could change himself. It said to take a pencil and paper and write down the assets one has. Use this list as a basis for developing a picture of the person one wants to become."

Ralph recounted how he did exactly that. "I pictured myself as an executive. I knew I'd have to know more, so I went to night school, studied, and nurtured the 'executive picture' in my mind. I even imagined the beautiful home I would have, the trips our family would take, and the way others would look at me as I walked to my private office in the morning.

"Things started changing. First a raise, then more responsibility. I know that I changed. Not overnight, but I could feel myself acting out the new pictures, the new self-image, that I had developed. I found that gradually everything became exactly the way I visualized it in my mind.

"That was only thirteen years ago. Today I have the beautiful home. We travel a lot. I have the private office.

"Don't underestimate the power of a mental image. Teach it. Write about it. Get people to develop a positive mental picture of what they want to become. It changed my life!"

CREATE YOUR OWN VISION

To manage the energy of thought to greater advantage is to bring into use the human being's unique gift—the visual imagination. It is quite possibly the least used of all the human talents, except by those who instinctively require its use in their daily work. The artist visualizes the picture before it goes on canvas. The pilot sees the landing in all its dimensions before the wheels touch the ground. The professional golfer pictures the swing and the shot before striking the ball.

You are empowered by your imagination. With your imagination you can construct the visions, the pictures, of what you want your life to be. Whatever those visions are, they will be realized in some fashion in the future.

You might say, "I've been doing that. I want to get ahead. I've been trying to lose weight, give up smoking, treat the kids better, get rid of my ulcers and headaches, and nothing much is happening. It doesn't work for me."

Doesn't it? Let's take a closer look. Sparked by ambition, a person thinks, "I'm going to work harder, overcome my laziness, learn more, and try saving money." That's the vision. What will be the state of being tomorrow? Simple—working harder, overcoming laziness, learning more, and trying to save money.

Another says, "For years I've tried everything to lose weight. I've gone to Super-Skinny, Pound-Pushers, Weight-Wizards, made bets with friends, been scared sleepless by my doctor, and my weight still is like a yo-yo. Goes up and down." That's the image, the vision, isn't it? What will be the state of being tomorrow? The same as it has been for all those yesterdays: struggling with weight, food, and calories—sometimes winning, sometimes losing.

The lesson is clear. Hold in your consciousness exactly what it is you want to be instead of what you are. That will mean a "paradigm shift," a change of the model, the perspective and image you have of yourself.

"That's not reality," you say. "It's just daydreaming. I'd be kidding myself." Would you? Human beings have the ability to envision who they would like to be and who they are capable of becoming. For many this lies dormant, never used. Why not use it to shape your existence and choose what you will become?

Fasten in your mind all the details of the success that you want. Know that you have already arrived. Give up the groping, hoping, someday wishes that perhaps it will happen to you.

Realize the love, depth, and richness of the relationships all about you. Envision yourself as a loved and loving person rather than lonely and bored, reaching out for someone who can make you happy.

Give up the self-concept of an overweight person jousting with extra pounds. Visualize that slender person within you waiting to emerge. Buy the clothing you will soon be wearing. Start being the person you want to be.

Stop believing that you're a fragile sack of flesh and bones, defenseless against sickness and age. Health and vitality are the natural and ageless qualities of the human being. Don't think of yourself as a sick person trying to get better. Claim your perfection now, and that will be your state of being tomorrow.

Remember, your vision today will be your state of being tomorrow. Decide the type of person you want to become, start collecting real pictures that portray that person. You can find them in magazines, newspapers, even snapshots you might take.

Visualize people who are living life the ways you want to live. Idols and heroes have long been known as the most significant influence on young peoples' lives. Tell me about your heroes and I'll tell you what kind of person you are.

Get pictures of the things you want to happen to you.

If you want to vacation in Tahiti, go to a travel agent and get a picture of Tahiti. If you want a new car, get a picture of the make and model you would like.

Hang all these visions, pictures, in the gallery of your mind. Realize the incredible significance of the two words *I am!* Whatever your hopes and dreams for the future, know that they are yours if you learn the power of "I am." Replace "I hope," "I would like," and all the other wistful wishes with "I am."

If it's success you want, know in your heart that you're already there. Picture all that success means to you—the home, security, financial independence, travel, and adventure. Pull it out of the musty dream stage and plant it firmly in your mind. Declare that you have that now. Use the words "I am!" That becomes your vision. It will, inevitably, become your state of being in the future.

If you're hoping to be successful someday, plugging along day after day, longing for more of the good things in life, that is your self-image. What, then, will be your state of being in the future? It will be hoping to be successful someday, plugging along day after day, longing for more of the good things in life.

Your vision today will be your state of being in the future. Life is meant to be lived with vigor, vitality, and good health. But only if you believe that is true. Let sickly negative thoughts creep into your mind, and they will surely shape your being in the future.

Indeed, it's not easy to declare your good health when your body is claiming illness. To say "I am complete, whole, healthy, and perfect" instead of thinking "I hope I get better" may seem hypocritical. But in a deeper sense it is quite the opposite. For one of the most potent forces of nature is the principle of healing and restoration. That perfect principle is within you working for your good.

Visualize it. Then care for your vision. Nurture it. Let it flourish. Let it become reality.

TWELVE

The Wonder of Words

OUR LIVES ARE SHAPED BY WORDS.

Stop, for a moment, and consider the wonder of words.
Perhaps they might be one of the most powerful, yet neglected,
forces available to direct your personal destiny.

Words give breath to thoughts. They enchant us—make us
laugh, or cry, or work, or play. Words are the mist of the mind drifting out to wrap others in whatever is our mood of the moment —
joy, sadness, hope, or despair.

Words build the castles of our lives. They are the tools of the
poet, the links of lovers, the playthings of children, the stepping-
stones of knowledge, the architects of society, the lights of enlightenment of that which is spiritual.

With words we build highways and buildings. With words
we produce and market our goods and services. With words we per-
petuate the knowledge and experience of humanity.

Words are the very special gift of God to the human being.
Words direct the course of civilization. They are responsible for
evolving humanity to its present state of development. Without
words we would still be groping about in herds, like animals, acting
out of instinct rather than intellect.

Our relationships are sensitized by words. They draw people

together or tear them apart. Words provide the nourishment of companionship.

Words are quite personal things, enabling us to grow, succeed, evolve into what we are capable of becoming. They shape our feelings about ourselves in relation to others.

But along with the power of words to work wonders also rests their tragic capabilities. They can destroy. They can cause misery and suffering.

Perhaps the significance of the spoken word is only a casual force compared to the profound effect of the unspoken word. The human being's thought processes are programmed by words. People think in words. And this mechanism may be one of the greatest marvels of life. For words that are run through the mind repetitiously inevitably become reality.

This phenomenon, when fully learned and controlled, can perhaps set aside many of the limitations of human existence. For example, words are being used to maintain and restore the health of the body. By a process termed biofeedback, individuals are taught how to use words in a relaxed state to eliminate all sorts of emotional and physical disorders.

All the disciplines and techniques, even the ancient meditative arts, all revolve about the mind's tendency to convert words into being.

You may have been using this power all of your life, except in a negative way. How many times, perhaps daily, do you feed limiting, restrictive words through your mind? "I can't get started." "I don't feel too peppy today." "It's a bad day for me."

Many of the negative words tumble through the mind so casually that they are not even noticed. But they surely are a reverse use of the power of the subconscious mind.

Medical science has undeniably proved that there is a language connection between your mind and your body. Your body believes the words and phrases it hears you utter, spoken aloud or silently. You will, infallibly, experience physically the thoughts that you verbalize, whether they are positive or negative, constructive or destructive.

When you say, "My supervisor gives me a pain in the neck," don't be surprised if you start needing aspirins.

"I can't live with this situation any more," may be a spontaneous reaction to inflamed feelings. But if the situation prevails, the body believes it is not supposed to keep living. The body does not know you didn't really mean what you said; you were just sort of venting.

Perhaps that is why many of the learned in the metaphysical sciences are projecting that we choose, consciously or unconsciously, when we will die. That's fairly heavy stuff and probably debatable. But why toy around with it? Why not just discipline the ways that you verbalize? Why not choose your aspirations of life and verbalize those?

WORDS CAN ENSLAVE

In Adventures In Attitudes, the participants analyze how words and phrases have had a negative impact on their attitudes. We call them "mind binders." Members write down and share their "mind binders." Here are some that are typical:

"I am afraid to speak in front of a group."
"I can't quit smoking."
"I can't remember people's names."
"I'll never be a wealthy person."

"I don't have much patience."

"I always get a cold when I get chilled."

"I have a poor memory."

"I don't have as much zip as I used to have."

"I can't get along with my neighbor."

"I get a headache when I don't get enough sleep."

"I'm not as smart as a lot of people."

"I can't lose weight because I can't stick to a diet."

"I can't get going in the morning."

"I don't like my job."

"I've got so much work to do. I don't know when I'll ever get it all done."

"I haven't felt too good lately."

"I need a vacation."

"I get nervous around strangers."

"I'm too old to change."

"I never had much of a chance."

"I don't really have any special talent."

"I can't think of things to talk about to people."

"The children get on my nerves."

"I can't save money."

"I'm self-conscious."

"I can't resist a piece of pie."

"I have bad luck."

"I worry a lot."

"I'm afraid to go up in a plane."

"I can't make up my mind what I want to do."

"I'm afraid I might get sick."

Do any of these sentences look familiar? Have you been telling yourself you are not as capable as others? Have you told yourself you are nervous, easily upset, irritated? Have you said you were not happy or not able to get ahead?

You were once thought to be mentally unhinged if you went about talking to yourself. Not anymore. It is now the acknowledged ritual to health and achievement. In fact, it has become an art and a science in itself.

You spend much of your day talking to yourself, verbalizing, running through scripts, many of which were created when you were a child. Adolescent scripts appear from time to time to limit and hold one back.

"She won't like me."

"I'm not ready yet."

"I don't know enough."

"She's a lot more popular than I am."

"It won't work for me."

"They will think I'm ridiculous."

"I'll never have time to get everything done."

"He's got a lot more going for him than I have."

Are you tearing yourself down or building yourself up? The primary block to people performing to the level of their potentials is self-interference, negative verbalizing. On the other hand, those people who are successful in their activities and relationships have the gift of accepting themselves, verbalizing positively, being their own best friends.

Remember James Allen's comparison of your mind to a garden? Just as the gardener cultivates the plot so may you "tend the garden of your mind, weeding out all the wrong, useless, and impure thoughts and cultivating toward perfection the flowers and fruit of right, useful, and pure thoughts."

You Can If You Think You Can

Consider replacing the words "I can't" in your thinking with "I can." A psychologist, Ben Sweetland, wrote an entire book titled *I Can.* In the opening pages he tells of an incident in one of his adult classes in a self-improvement course:

"A man, in his late fifties, attended regularly, hoping that through the messages I was giving, he would find the magic thought which would elevate him to a place where he could support his wife, instead of being supported by her.

"The job he had held for years came to an end and in trying to find another one, he was constantly confronted with the statement: 'You're too old.'

"Week after week, Bill Jones (we'll call him) arrived for the lecture with an expectant look on his face, but would leave with the feeling that his pursuit of an answer to his problem had been fruitless.

"There was an exception to this weekly routine—something happened. Ending a lecture and approaching Bill—instead of seeing his long drawn face—there was an expression of great exuberance. 'I've got the answer!' he exclaimed with a tone of actual excitement. Naturally I was happy—and eager to learn just what it was that turned the tide from depression to ecstasy.

"Bill took me to the chair where he had been sitting and pointed to a visible portion of an electric sign which was mounted on the top of a building several blocks away. The word 'American' was part of the wording of the sign—and where Bill sat—he could see but the last four letters, I CAN.

"'There's the answer to my problem, Ben,' he said with excitement. 'Up to now I have been thinking in terms of "I Can't,"' and continuing said, 'all evening those four letters have been glaring at me—as though intended as a message from above especially for me.'

" 'I CAN, Ben,' Bill declared, 'and tomorrow I am going to prove it.' "

Ben Sweetland then devotes his book to describing how one's life can be changed by saying "I can!" to life instead of "I can't."

Try it. Look in a mirror. Remind yourself of your strengths and resource. Say, "I love you," to that face you see. Why not? That's who you'll be with for the rest of your life. Verbalize all the things you can do rather than what you can't do.

A new era of human awareness has dawned, radiant with hope and wonder. Encased within your being is the most awesome mechanism in the universe. Explosive with unknown miracles, words repeated silently with conviction and authority will be transformed into reality.

So value words. Hold them in esteem. They shape your thinking. They are the garments of your thoughts. They make the portals of your mind galleries of splendor or closets of wretchedness. They are the guideposts of your journey through life which will lead you to fields of abundance or swamps of despair.

Practice verbalizing positively as a step toward personal empowerment.

A few words, assembled with meaning, can be beacons of light in millions of lives, inspiring hope, kindness, and self-confidence. Such was a message that sprung into being more than a century ago from an unknown origin.

"I shall pass through this world but once. Any good, therefore, that I can do, or any kindness that I can show to any human being, let me do it now. Let me not defer nor neglect it, for I shall not pass this way again."

This quotation, passed on from generation to generation through books, magazines, sermons, seminars, and friend-to-friend, has caused millions to treat others with more kindness and respect. King George V was known to have copied the epic by hand and kept it on his desk.

"Any good that I can do, or any kindness that I can show to any human being, let me do it now." This has been a prescription for happiness by all those remembered for their contributions to human wholeness —Florence Nightingale, Dale Carnegie, Emily Dickinson, Albert Schweitzer…the list is endless.

Emile Coué, the psychotherapist, worked miracles with French peasants who came to his clinic for help. The lame, the sick, and the suffering were cured. His methods were easily understood and practiced. He originated, for instance, the following sentence and suggested it be repeated dozens of times each day: "Every day, in every way, I am getting better and better."

Coué was shocked when he came to America to find that he was almost totally ineffective. A comparison of those he treated explained why. The French peasant, living plainly close to the soil, was believing, receptive, and unsuspecting. The American mind, to the contrary, was calcified by complex, hurried, and organization-oriented living. Imaginations were stifled by conformity; new concepts were viewed skeptically with logic; visions were cloaked with segmented theory.

Is there a lesson here? Should we free our minds from self-imposed bondage? Are we really intellectually superior and sophisticated or have our egos draped our minds with shrouds of cerebral deceptions?

Of one reality you can be certain. Words repeated with authority and conviction can have a profound effect on your life and those around you. They can be spring boards for your personal empowerment.

Verbalize. Verbalize hourly, daily, weekly with positive affirmations.

You have just been given two examples.

"Any good that I can do, or any kindness that I can show to any human being, let me do it now, for I shall not pass this way again."

"Every day, in every way, I'm getting better and better." Coué had impressive results by suggesting to French mothers that they breath those words into the ears of their children. Could we follow such earthly advice gently reminding our children of some of the more fundamental values of life?

USE AFFIRMATIONS

In our program, Adventures In Attitudes, we emphasize the use of affirmations. Feedback from those completing the program has indicated an impressive long-lasting influence on many lives.

Being involved with the use of affirmations, several precepts have evolved that contribute to their effectiveness.

1.) Keep your affirmations short, preferably single sentences that are easily remembered. Repeated often, they become habitual responses to situations, feelings, and events. If your mind is busy creating, searching for words, it is not being galvanized with affirmation empowerment. Printing an affirmation on the back of a 3" x 5" or business card has been beneficial.

2.) Make declarations of desired positive characteristics rather than the negative millstones you feel should be eliminated. If you are making a statement that you are trying to rid yourself of baggage like guilt, criticism, self-destruction, inferiority, anger and such, you are giving power and energy to those parasites. You are actually adding fuel to that which you are trying to heal. So "that which you greatly fear will come upon you."

Remember, during your waking moments, a thought can never be removed, only replaced. Positive affirmations are like turning on a light in a dark room. The darkness vanishes doesn't it? Don't be concerned about the shadows in your mind! They will disappear with the radiance of positive statements.

There is one exception. If you are ready to devote a quiet time to your attitude enrichment you might start by stating: "I release all thoughts of confusion, tension, anxiety, and irritation to clear my mind for wholesome nourishment. I am open, relaxed, and receptive."

3.) Use words like "I am" and "I can," focusing on the present rather than the past or future. Your passion for today will displace the burdens of yesterday or the worries of tomorrow.

4.) Affirmations are the wings that skywrite messages on your mind. Personalize them. Create them as extensions of your visualizations, your self-image.

5.) These are not hard and fast rules, only suggested guidelines. Work with your affirmations. You will experience an empowering effect after a short time, even a couple weeks. If you find an affirmation that works for you, keep it. If it doesn't, let it go.

That idea, indeed, may be applied to any compartment of your life. If you find something that works for you, hang on to it; if you find something that doesn't work, let it go.

Here are typical affirmations that might be helpful in constructing your own.

SELF-ESTEEM

You are like a snowflake; no two are alike. You are a unique, very special expression of life. Accept yourself. Like yourself. Praise yourself. Dwell on your strengths, abilities, potentials. Build your self-esteem.

1.) There is a power and splendor within me that surpasses my understanding, yet is what I am.

2.) I am empowered by my courage, strength, and optimism.

3.) Every day I grow stronger in mind, body, and spirit.

4.) I have an unlimited capacity for peace, poise, power, and perfection.

5.) I am inspired, enthused, and excited about my life's opportunities.

6.) My words have power to create, guide, and determine my life's potentials.

7.) I cherish today's moments to think, feel, and celebrate the wonder of my life.

8.) I believe in myself, my abilities, my uniqueness, my gifts of life.

PERSONAL GROWTH

1.) I welcome the mystery and magic of change and growth. I allow it to happen easily and harmoniously.

2.) Every day in every way I am becoming better and better.

3.) I am led to where my talents and abilities will be used to their greatest advantage.

4.) Every day I am being reborn into someone more magnificent than I have ever been before.

5.) I am energized by my dreams, visions, and excitement for life.

6.) I am refreshed, nourished, and enthused by my aspirations and expectations.

7.) I grow in understanding and wisdom by the differences I experience with others.

INTERACTION WITH OTHERS

1.) Any good that I can do, or any kindness that I can show another, I will do it now.

2.) I view all others as potential teachers from whom I can learn.

3.) I encourage, comfort, and support others.

4.) I will do unto others as I would have them do unto me.

5.) My words and actions will reflect my care and understanding of others.

6.) I know that my freedom is dependent on giving others theirs.

7.) I act with patience, empathy and love in my relationships.

8.) I rejoice in the happiness and success of those around me.

9.) Harmony, peace, unity, and love prevail in my home.

10.) I understand myself as I seek to understand others.

11.) I grow in my wholeness by adding to that of my beloved.

12.) I attract and am surrounded by those who inspire, enthuse, and sustain me.

13.) I look for and see greatness and good in others.

14.) I celebrate others' success, achievements, and prosperity.

15.) My life is enriched by the love and presence of family and friends.

16.) I treasure the beauty and goodness I see in my loved ones.

DAILY ACTIVITY

The ways that you spend your day can be made meaningful and satisfying with affirmations. All work is centered on service to others. That service performed with diligence and pride will inevitably lead to rewards of prosperity, abundance, and fulfillment. If your activity is committed to caring for others or a home, know that you are wearing the crown of life's deepest purpose.

1.) There is an infinite supply and abundance in the universe that will flow to me in response to my service.

2.) My daily activity is a vehicle for my vision, strength, and energy.

3.) Today, my work will express life's noblest meaning of service to others.

4.) I serve with enthusiasm, joy, and humility.

5.) I am a leader and teacher at home and at work for I look behind me and see others following me.

6.) I share my efforts, talents, and resources with others.

7.) I encourage others to express their ideas, opinions, and insight.

8.) This day will be spent devoted to the highest and best use of my human qualities.

9.) I have a growing awareness of my boundless potential, success, and opportunities to serve.

10.) My focus is centered on serving, satisfying, and succeeding.

HEALTH

Positive affirmations will help sustain a healthy body because they maintain a healthy mind. They build faith in the enormous healing power of the body and its ability to resist sickness and disease.

Positive affirmations of health, healing, and restoration will dilute the devastating influences of fear, worry, and symptoms of physical malfunctions.

1.) Every cell of my body is filled with glowing health and vitality.

2.) Healing energy is constantly renewing, rebuilding, restoring, and maintaining my body in perfect health.

3.) I am filled with life-giving energy, health, and wholeness.

4.) My body functions with preordained order, harmony, and balance.

5.) I look beyond the illusions of sickness and know that there is only one law of healing working within me, becoming more effective with my positive declarations.

We have been considering the empowering characteristics of visualizing and verbalizing. Those are tools for managing your mind. A suggestion—don't hold the reins too tight. Relax. Be at peace.

There is a quaint childish quality resting within your soul that resists growing up. It delights in games, silly times, and pretending. In the pressures of the adult world with problems, ambitions, and the frantic pursuit of material gadgetry, the child often becomes submerged, rendered immobile. With that, some of the lighter and brighter joys of life sink into oblivion.

Cherish your child. Let it play. Let it daydream. Let it dance. Let it look about you with its infant curiosity and poke and push and squeeze and hug and taste and learn.

Set your marvelous child free to romp about in the meadows of your imagination, having fun with people and flowers and animals. Allow it to be spontaneous and impulsive at times, taking you where it will.

Enjoying the child can be risky. Climbing a mountain, skydiving, exploring unknown pathways of life, although exhilarating, can be hazardous. But, while there is an elf-child in your soul, there is also an adult who will step in and act as the protector, the guardian.

Look within. You will discover, not just one person, but many, all of different ages and dispositions. Such is the mysticism of life. It is also wholeness.

THIRTEEN

Dealing With Feelings

THE CONCUSSION OF A CLANGING ALARM CLOCK IS JOSTLING YOUR SLEEP-DRENCHED MIND. "Uhhh—I'd give my Christmas bonus for just another 10 minutes," you think. But, no. There's a meeting and this is Thursday. Gobs of debris must be cleared out before the weekend. Coffee will help. Two cups later you find it does. The pulse is quicker. The brain is clear. All systems are on go.

Except for the traffic. Road repairs have imprisoned you in a line of cars sentencing you to a minimum 15-minute delay. "I should have gone the other way. Is it too late? Can I hit the shoulder and pass the cars ahead? What are they holding things up for? They can let those cars get around that grader! What will the others think when I drag in 15 minutes late?" Frantic thoughts turn on more adrenaline.

The meeting doesn't do anything to slow things down. In between sips of coffee you try to bat down some of the resistance to your viewpoint. Not enough time.

The get-together breaks up. But not the pattern of activity. More problems. More rush. More traffic. The stomach feels like a clenched fist. Sweaty palms, throbbing head and frustration are all clamoring for a tranquilizer and a quiet evening of TV.

But there are just a couple little decisions that must be made before dinner. Like where will we spend next year's vacation? And

Alfred has a learning problem, so shall we move him to a special school? And Jennifer does not seem happy at that daycare center. Shall we talk about that? Incidentally, with both of us working, things don't seem to be the same between us. And remember, Aunt Bertha and Uncle Bill are coming to visit for a few days. Wouldn't it be nice to get a new car before they got here?

There is no longer any appetite or hope for a peaceful evening. Simple anxiety and tension have been replaced by a kind of smoldering rage. The inner mechanism is in full battle posture, ready to defend you against the world, its people, and the pits into which you have been thrust. You are experiencing the bubonic plague of the 20th century—stress.

Forget about cholesterol, asbestos fibers, sugar, and air clogged with carbon dioxide. The number one killer today is stress. Endured over a period of time, this hoarded pressure must find a release. Ulcers, nervous breakdowns, heart attacks, high blood pressure, even cancer are a few of the outlets the body finds. Or the relief could be sought in compulsive eating, marriage splits, temper tantrums, and addictions. These can all be triggered by stress.

The researchers in the areas of religion, science, and human behavior are targeting stress. What is being discovered is little more than your common sense tells you, but that you don't want to admit.

For instance, you cause your own stress. Now, that's hard to digest along with your Valium. It's that cockeyed boss, stains on the carpeting, kids screaming, weeds in the rose bushes, too much to do and too little time to do it that's wrenching your nervous system. Nope. They're not what's doing it. It's your reactions to all those things that creates any stress you feel.

You bring a gang of gremlins into your life and then give

them the power to play tug-of-war with your nerves. Like most other problems, stress is shaped only in the mind.

To you, conquering the mountain of insurmountable problems in your life may be like climbing Mt. Everest. To another, coping with the same batch of sticklers would seem like a stroll around the block. It's a matter of personal attitude. In a way, that's promising. Because what is created by thought can be taken apart the same way. You can control stress by learning to manage your attitudes.

"Ah! Sweet relief!" You might say, "now I have the secret."

Almost. But not quite. Because in the midst of all the palpitations, tension, and anxiety you discover you can't quiet them by thought alone. You are verifying a psychological fact. You cannot, by your willpower, control your emotions.

When there is a contest between your will and your emotions, the emotions will win, hands down, nine out of ten times. Let's try an example. Here is a plank, 20 feet long and a foot wide, resting on the ground. Can you walk on top of it from one end to the other? "Of course," you reply as you skip along without even looking down.

Will you do it again for a vacation in Tahiti? "Easy," you reply as you start toward the board. But, hold on! There's going to be a slight change. This time the plank is going to be extended from the top of a building fifty stories in the air. Are your feelings going to hold you back from something your willpower knows you can do? Probably. Your stomach quivers and your heart bumps up somewhere near your tonsils just thinking about it.

Are the dare-devils, tight-rope walkers, trapeze artists, and stunt performers immune from fear and apprehension? Of course not. They have learned to subdue such shackling emotions. How?

By practice. By gradually acting out what they want to become. Confidence gradually triumphs over the hobgoblins of fright.

So you can not, by your will, manipulate your feelings. But you can, by your will, control your actions. You tend to feel the way that you act.

FEELING FOLLOWS ACTION

Aha! That's the real secret! That's the antidote to stress.

If you act calm, you tend to feel calm.

If you act peacefully, you tend to feel peaceful.

If you act patiently, you tend to feel patient.

If you act relaxed, you tend to feel relaxed.

If you act with quietness and serenity, the temperature of your stress slides down.

It gets better! If you act happy, you feel happy.

If you act successful, you will feel successful.

If you act with enthusiasm, you will feel enthusiastic.

"Suit the action to the word, the word to the action," advised Shakespeare in Hamlet.

In exploring the wonders of your mind, visualize, yes, and verbalize, yes, but then practice the final step—vitalize. Vitalize means "give life to."

Giving life to your images and affirmations through your actions is to ignite them with emotion. Your nerve fibers act like little switches. Where there is no emotion, the switches are closed and lifeless. But when there is emotion the switches open, become connected, and things start happening!

Sometimes good; sometimes bad.

There are those lovely, wondrous emotions that you want to flourish in your life—love, happiness, excitement, joy, cheer—the

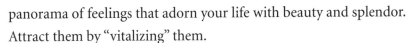

panorama of feelings that adorn your life with beauty and splendor. Attract them by "vitalizing" them.

But there are also the feelings that might plague you—depression, anger, grief, fear, anguish—to name a few.

They, too, can be moderated by vitalizing their opposites—supported by visualizing and affirmations.

William James, our dean of American psychologists, would agree. He wrote:

> *"We need only in cold-blood to act as if the thing in question were real and it will infallibly end by growing into such a connection with our life that it will become real!"*

Admittedly, your feelings are not only caused by actions but also by reactions. If you are betrayed by a loved one, you will likely feel anger and resentment. Or it's a sunny day; you are having lunch with a dear friend. You get to work and are greeted with a few compliments and a raise in pay. You feel elated, warm, and satisfied.

So your emotions react to the ups and downs of your daily activities. But why abandon your feelings entirely to the whims and wherefores of people and circumstances? You need not be a victim or a captive of the roller-coasters of happenstance. You can be liberated by practicing strategies that provide choices and put you in charge of your life.

A GIFT FOR YOU

Here is a gift you can hold close to your heart and will become more precious with use. It is an affirmation that thousands have received who have attended Adventures In Attitudes; many testify it is one of the most commonly recalled nuggets of the program.

"I can't help the way I feel right now, but I can help the way I think and act."

I'll applaud those words as loud and long as many others; whenever my emotions are in an upheaval and seem to be stamping beyond control, I repeat this affirmation.

My forty-year-old son, Jim, is finely tuned emotionally, a splendid asset, really, but one that needs mature self-monitoring. He recently told me, "Dad, I still use that phrase, 'I can't help the way I feel right now, but I can help the way I think and act.'"

Jim has trophy-winning skills building and racing motorcycles. He thrills to the excitement and competition of the national events. But not on freeways. When he is on his Harley and an auto driver thoughtlessly or deliberately threatens his safety, an emotional response is triggered. Jim has learned that, "I can help the way I think and act," will prevent a possible vital confrontation.

We're all driving our Harleys, aren't we? But they weigh a little more and have four wheels. We climb into them, start them rolling and are immediately threatened, intimidated, and endangered by people whose sanity and maturity is somehow lost when their egos and competitive urges are expressed in a couple tons of moving machinery. That is when you will cherish this gift: "I can't help the way I feel right now, but I can help the way I think and act."

DEALING WITH ANGER

Our highways and byways are filled with angry people. But driving vehicles is not the only cause of the flare-ups. There are many others.

Look behind anger and you will find a suffering person, one who is in pain. In the ignorance fostered by rage, it is believed that the only way to be relieved of the inner turmoil of anger is to hurt another. Therein lies the cause of violence, torment, killing, beating, and such. These are the embers of anger blown into a blaze by inner rage.

Why? Why let anger dictate your actions? And you say, "I can't help it. I have a quick temper. I don't think I can keep from being angry." You're right. If you have convinced yourself that you cannot control anger then that affirmative belief is your reality.

Try reversing your thinking. At the next spark that threatens to touch off that short fuse, say to yourself, "I can't help the way I feel right now, but I can help the way I think and act. I will stop being angry. My anger is destructive. It destroys me. It chews away at my wholeness, my well-being. It tears apart my love, the essence of my soul. It drives thorns into my relationships."

Anger is not natural. It is unnatural. Why make yourself and others miserable by hanging on to anger and trying to justify it? Let it go. Stop being angry.

The modern ideas about anger are generally fostered and nourished by an anger industry that assumes that behind every tranquil soul is a furious being screaming to get out. So it is believed that to discharge one's feelings by "letting it all hang out" or to "blow off steam" by arguing, shouting, hitting, or working off feelings will rid one of the vials of wrath.

But Carol Tavris, author of *Anger: The Misunderstood Emotion*, disagrees. All it does is raise the noise level of one's life and does little to solve any problems. She points out that people giving vent to their anger only get angrier, not less angry. Besides, there are a lot of hurt feelings by the recipients of rage.

She probes all the destructive effects of "ventilating" anger in marital relationships—outbursts, recriminations, crying, and critical reactions. Acting angry doesn't release it; you're only rehearsing it. Evidence indicates that men expressing anger are more prone to heart disease. A batch of other data is unveiled, all of it suggesting that anger expressed contributes nothing positive to your health, relationships, or career.

If you do feel angry, Tavris suggests, the best antidote is still "count to 10." Just let it go away.

An article some time ago in *Psychology Today* titled "Anger Defused," stated: "There's little evidence that suppressing anger is dangerous to health. In fact, studies show that 'getting it off your chest' only makes you angrier."

These notions are not really new.

Nearly 2,000 years ago a Greek slave, Epictetus, was freed by his master and taught philosophy in Rome. Later he was expelled from Rome, perhaps for doctrines such as this: "Whenever you are angry, be assured that it is not only a present evil, but that you have increased a habit."

Such ideas were not popular then nor now. For people hang on to their anger, justifying the reasons for feeling the way they do. Indeed, it is a common belief that the only way to get rid of anger is to show it.

Why do they say that by expressing anger you get rid of it, but when expressing love you acquire more of it?

The truth is that you tend to feel emotion more frequently as it is expressed. The illusion that a negative emotion like anger, hate, or hostility is eliminated by its demonstration is because any emotion that is expressed leaves one feeling relieved and to an extent, satisfied. There is a sense of comfort by showing prejudice, rage, vengeance, or grief as well as love, happiness, joy, and pride.

Also existing is a tendency of the human organism to return and repeat those forms of behavior that provide satisfaction. If it is anger, then there is an inner urge to be angry. If it's love, then there is an inclination to feel love. This is the way habits and addictions are formed.

An individual has a natural motivation to feel good. So the attraction of the human mechanism is to repeat the process that produced the good feeling. If that was anger, then on occasion, an instinctive impulse arises to be drawn into the script that induced anger. As that role is learned and a part of the behavior pattern, it becomes more spontaneous and habitual, just as love becomes easier and easier to feel when demonstrated openly and frequently.

Some say that relationships, at times, must go through a dialogue of irritation. That's just a viewpoint, one, perhaps, that is only a justification for the continued hostility or rage that persists.

Deep, rich relationships are only bonded by love, harmony, and synergism. Anger doesn't make a good relationship better. Any time such a union is ruptured by anger and blame, it never quite gets back to where it was. Every wedge of wrath driven into a really fine relationship restricts it from its ultimate potential.

Where does all this take us? Emotions must be examined. What are they doing to one's life? What are the effects on others? Obviously anger gets negative reactions. No long-range therapeutic or beneficial emotional results are derived by forming habits of showing ill temper.

This does not mean that anger should not be felt. Nor should it be buried to come forth another day in some unhealthy manner. Look behind the anger and you will find meaning, maybe hurt. For anger is often defensive, a protective shield from harm or emotional pain.

Don't suppress the embers of rage, but don't allow them to spring into flame and take over your life. Such feelings can be managed. Talking and thinking about your anger is different from the anger talking and thinking for itself.

At times you must go through suffering to find your peace. When intense emotional upheavals are experienced, listen to them. They may be telling you to leave a part of your life that is waiting to be shed.

If you find the fuse getting shorter and shorter in a job, it may be a sign that you're due for a career change. When lingering feelings of impatience and anger persist after being with certain people, these could be cues that your life would run better without these particular associations.

If a relationship needs anger to keep it glued together, either as therapy for the one showing anger or martyrdom for the one absorbing it, then it's a symptom of sickness. One may well question the wisdom of clinging to such a link. Such omens could indicate a need to grow, to fly on to a more mature companionship.

Visualize, Verbalize, Vitalize

Vitalize. Stay in control of your actions, for they will surely influence your emotions. Your feelings will react to your thoughts and actions. Say, "I can't help the way I feel right now, but I can help the way I think and act."

If your feelings are acting like they're eating hot peppers, physical activity might soothe and comfort. Take a walk, chase squirrels, clean a closet, wash the car, weed the garden, scrub the bathroom floor. But don't act crazy. All you will be doing is adding guilt to your anger.

Visualize, verbalize, and vitalize like my middle-aged friend, Denny, a successful business executive. We were discussing these strategies of self-empowerment at lunch one day. He told me, "I have not been angry during the last five years. Five years ago I realized that I could not be angry and be healthy. The two didn't go together. Anger was taking away a lot of the things I wanted in life. I was paying a heavy price to be angry. I knew of no other way to rid myself of that self-destruction except to simply stop being angry.

"Every day I get up and tell myself 'Don't be angry today!' That includes the way I look at myself; I stopped being angry with me. I started forgiving myself, concentrating on strengths instead of weaknesses. Taking anger out of my life left quite a space. A lot of positive things have rushed in to fill that void. Ridding myself of anger has changed my life."

WORKING THROUGH HIGHS AND LOWS

How do we deal with the less volatile emotions? How about our moods? Moods are the playmates of life. They frolic. They pout. They are joy and peace. Or they can be anxiety, depression, or despair.

Moods react. They are sensitive to the circumstances and events of life. But they sometimes seem to give birth to themselves, for no apparent reason, in the womb of the mind. Moods are a sizable chunk of your life; when they are playful and spirited, bringing moments of happiness and joy, they are taken for granted. But when they are burdensome and lethargic, causing dullness or anguish, they become a dilemma.

So how do you deal with the unpleasant moods—the ones that appear from nowhere that cast a cloud on the hours of the day? Let's think about that. Let's think about the way we think about moods.

Would it make a difference if we stop putting labels like "bad," "awful," or "not in a good" mood? Look at moods as friends.

They enable you to experience the full panorama of life. They are the rhythm and symphony of life. But to know them as the highs you must also experience the lows.

You are never the same, although you may seem to be; you are constantly being transformed, renewed, and changed. The very nature of life is one of reaching out, becoming what you are capable of becoming; you are subtly growing, learning, adjusting, and creating. Moods provide the incubation for that process. They are as much a part of your emotional growth as the food that nourishes your body. Without moods the evolution of your life would be stifled.

So let's stop thinking about moods as being ugly and a departure from the nicer, more lovely self. Stop beating them, feeling guilty, or bearing them as the unexplainable loads of life. Stop trying to suppress them with an upper or a downer. Stop drowning them with booze or suffocating them with bonbons.

Be kind to your mood, whatever it is. Treat it gently. Let it tip-toe around in your mind and emotions and take you where it will. Realize that your mind needs these spaces to prepare you for transitions ahead.

Don't panic. Don't let your mind trick you into believing the mood has any permanence. Know that "this too shall pass away."

Don't interfere with the little known purpose and course of your moods. Open your mind; let them exist.

You can, however, tenderly guide them with some well-chosen words and actions. Visualize, verbalize, vitalize. We have some simple devices used in Adventures In Attitudes that remind the participant of these processes. Cards are used imprinted with the words, "I AM," "I CAN," and "I WILL." I encourage you to obtain some 3" x 5" cards and make your own.

Those simple artless cards have had an amazing effect on many lives when displayed in the home, office, or car.

Try, also, to be more specific in the characteristic you want to vitalize. For instance, print "PATIENCE" on cards and put them in places where you see them often.

Lew, a grisly, short-tempered business executive said, "That PATIENCE card has turned my whole day around. I put one on the visor of my car and start for work five minutes earlier. I get to the office relaxed instead of all beat and pumped up by the traffic demons. Besides, I've become the most courteous driver on the highway."

Countless numbers of lives could be saved if auto manufacturers were required to imprint "PATIENCE" on the visors of every car.

Vitalize! Give life to what you want to become by your actions. Ralph Waldo Emerson advised: "He who does the thing has the power; he who does not do the thing has not the power."

Socrates stated: "Study to be what you wish to seem." Study to be the person you wish to appear. Visualize that person; then verbalize being that person; then vitalize, bring life to that person, through your actions.

That, then, is the sixth assignment for becoming personally empowered: "Visualize, Verbalize, Vitalize."

ASSIGNMENT NUMBER SEVEN

"Learn to Learn"

FOURTEEN

Learn to Learn

> *"I'm always ready to learn, although
> I do not always like being taught."*
> —Winston Churchill

"LEARN TO LEARN" IS THE SEVENTH ASSIGNMENT FOR PERSONAL EMPOWERMENT. What you are taught can bind you; what you learn can free you. Learn to learn. Escape from self-inflicted restrictions.

You start out in life learning how to learn. You're curious. You poke, push, break, tear apart, wobble around, fall down, get up, knock over the flower pot, put your finger on a hot stove, spit out food you don't like, and take risks, exploring the world about you— always trying, trying, trying.

Then you attend school. That triggers a process that continues long into your adult life. You are trained to be taught.

Schools teach how to memorize, not how to think.

Deeper issues are not probed in formal schooling. Character. Integrity of the soul. Selective perception. Problem-solving. Self-esteem. Getting along with others. Personal development. Attitude enrichment. Those are a few of the powerful forces of life that are neglected by the urgency of cybernating information.

That's the educational system. It provides an incredible amount of knowledge about a vast array of subjects. Except the one that is most important—you. Your years of education are finished with, perhaps, more questions than there are answers about your life and what to do with it.

When you are an adult, the tribes of which you are a member may follow the same rituals of teaching. You are taught to be taught, not to learn how to learn. There is, in fact, a risk implied by going beyond the prescribed boundaries and thinking for yourself.

Each religion, for instance, beholds itself as the delineator of God. To stray from its doctrine is to stray from God.

The corporation clones the employees to its culture, policies, and procedures. Some call it "industrial momism." Disagreement may provoke failure.

Should you depart from the institutions? Are they wrong? No. To be cradled within them is to be secure, anchored in place, seeded in fertile soil that can nourish growth. But from the nests of safeness, look down and within. You will probably find a wincing enigma of who you are and what you can become. Know that there is more, much more to life than is being taught. There is a potential, an unlimited vista beyond the institutions, implanted belief systems, educational processes and training programs. It rests in here, your soul, not out there. You are a miracle, a spiritual being templed in a physical body. Do not allow the learning skills that are inherently frolicking to unravel the mysteries of life become numbed and withered by outside forces. Learn to learn.

That might mean finding the curious little child within who, many forgotten years ago, spent all day groping, risking, growing, discovering unknown abilities. Let's start with the following axioms.

LESSONS OF LIFE

1. You will learn only what you want to learn, when you want to learn it.

2. All events, however trivial, are lessons. Even those events labeled as mistakes, failures, or problems are only lessons.

3. All lessons, properly learned, will lead to your spiritual growth.

4. Lessons are gifts of life. A lesson will be repeated until it is learned. When it is learned you can then go on to the next lesson.

5. The answers to all your questions of what you will become rest within. "Look well into thyself; there is a source which will always spring up if thou wilt always search there." —Marcus Aurelius.

6. Learn to learn, for that is the pathway to enlightenment and personal empowerment.

How do you learn to learn? Sorry. I can't answer that. No one can. Like the duckling breaking from the shell, you must do that yourself. The discovery comes from your aspiration, your desire to learn.

We can however, probe the assignment together. I can share my experiences, my perspectives, and perhaps they will influence your awareness. And reactions.

In my classes of Adventures In Attitudes, we spent time discussing learning to learn. There seemed to be agreement that the practice starts with a question.

The human mind works very much like a computer. Feed it a question and it will search until it finds an answer. We were told this long before the age of the computer. "Ask, and it will be given you; seek, and you will find; knock, and it will be opened to you."

Questions open the mind like the petals of a flower. The mind becomes receptive to the light of lessons. Learn to ask questions. As you long for better answers, ask better questions. Those are important. Look behind the words for unwritten meanings. Your meanings. Your reactions. If you find yourself disagreeing, that does not make the words any less useful. You often learn more in disagreement than you do in agreement.

Participants in my classes analyzed and experienced a variety of questions. Typical of the ones more favored were questions like these:

"What is the meaning of this?"

"Why?"

"What goes on here?"

"What is the lesson to be learned?"

We named such questions "Mind motivators." They stirred the mind to inquire, examine, ask. Practice the art of questioning. Nurture it. Let it empower you. Look beyond the lecture, the books, the arrangement of the stars, the month in which you were born, the latest revelation by the tabloids, or the dire predictions of the clairvoyant. Open your mind with questions. Learn to learn.

CAUSE AND EFFECT

All events have a cause and an effect. That's karma. Identifying the karma of episodes can lead to some of the more significant lessons of life. Learning to ascertain karma is a resource, a talent. Mind motivators help.

There is the story of the fellow who trained a flea to jump on command.

Then, day by day, he pulled out one of the flea's legs. Every time a leg was removed, the insect had more difficulty jumping. When the last leg was finally gone, the fellow said, "Jump!" The flea, of course, couldn't move.

"This simply shows that when you remove all of the flea's legs, the flea becomes deaf," the guy explained.

Wrong karma. Wrong lesson. Learn further.

One of my class members told of an incident involving a young juvenile caught several times stealing food. Why would he steal? He was subjected to psychological evaluations and testing. Several conclusions were drawn based on behavioral characteristics.

But the arresting police officer came up with the right one. The boy was hungry. Right karma. Right lesson.

George A. Miller, past president of the American Psychological Association stated: "The mind is a mismatch detector. It's easier for us to see what is wrong than to see what is right."

"Failure." "Wrong." "Bad." "Mistake." These are all labels put on events that confuse the karma.

A fable in oriental folklore tells about a farmer wandering along a country road looking anxiously at the road before him. A neighbor saw him and asked, "Is something troubling you, my friend?"

"My horse ran away," the farmer relied.

"Oh, that's too bad!" the neighbor exclaimed.

"Is it?" the farmer responded.

The next day the two met again. "Did you find your horse?" the neighbor inquired.

"Yes," the farmer replied.

"Oh, that's good!" the neighbor said.

"Is it?" the farmer uttered.

The next day they met again. "How is your horse?" asked the neighbor.

"A bit wild," the farmer mentioned. "He threw my son and my son broke his leg."

"Oh, that's too bad." the neighbor said.

"Is it?" the farmer asked.

The next time they met, the country had gone to war. The farmer explained that all young men were drafted into the army. His son was exempt because of this broken leg.

It is a quaint little anecdote with the rather profound philosophy that events in life are only good or bad according to one's perspective.

How do you deal with your "horses that run away"?

Every incident, every experience, every trifling episode, links together to evolve into greater meaning. Each is a cause for a trailing effect. Knowing that, one can choose what those effects will be.

Who is to say that the lost sale, a sniffly nose, flat tire, or irritating rebuke are incidents that must be labeled as "too bad"?

Perhaps the lost sale may be a learning experience that will gain ten others. Or it might lead to an extra measure of determination with far greater rewards than just the single sale.

Maybe the sniffly nose prompts a few hours of rest when a good book is read or a bright idea is generated. Or it might be only a gentle reminder that glowing health is, indeed, a blessing that needs mental and physical nourishment.

The flat tire only disabled the auto for a time. How fortunate that it is not a blowout that could cause a serious accident. Or was it the opportunity to realize the goodness of others when a stranger stopped and offered to help?

That irritating rebuke may have a splinter of justification. There are other ways to respond other than to attack or defend.

Those two are the customary responses, aren't they? Either the other person must be attacked or the rebuke must be proved untrue. Neither works.

How about listening, thanking the other, and then pondering on the critical remark for a time? If it has no validity, then merely forgive and forget. On the other hand, there may be an objective in sight that can lead to substantial personal growth.

Most important, do not look back with remorse and self-pity. A prominent psychologist recently said that the majority of his patients would not be in his office if they could avoid the words, "What if…"

If they were to stop looking back and creating worry, sorrow and "poor me" pictures with their illusions of "what if," then they would not be mired in their psychological swamps of despair.

So much for those events that one might evaluate like the farmer's neighbor by saying, "Oh, that's too bad."

How about the incident which might be viewed by exclaiming, "Oh that's good!"

The farmer's comment, "Is it?" might be worth considering. Much can be learned by dealing with the good happenings in life. Are they shared? Are they stepping stones to more significant events? Are they accepted with humility and thankfulness?

Anyone can handle failure. Millions do it day after day. But it requires remarkable wisdom, maturity, and unselfishness to wear the cloaks of success. Particularly challenging when a certain measure of success is achieved is not to view success as a parking lot for lethargy and complacency.

William Shakespeare expressed it another way when he wrote:

"Nothing is good or bad, but thinking makes it so."

Learn to learn, karma. Mind motivators. Review, again, our "Lessons of life."

1. You will learn only what you want to learn when you want to learn it.

2. All events, however trivial, are lessons—even those labeled as mistakes, failures, or problems are only lessons.

3. All lessons, properly learned, will lead to your spiritual growth.

4. Lessons are gifts of life. A lesson will be repeated until it is learned. When it is learned you can then go on to the next lesson.

5. The answers to all your questions of what you will become rest within. *"Look well into thyself; there is a source which will always spring up if thou wilt always search there."*

—*Marcus Aurelius*

6. Learn to learn for that is the pathway to enlightenment and personal empowerment.

LESSONS ARE OFTEN OVERLOOKED

Lessons must be presented again and again because the events in which the lessons are encased are passed by, ignored. Bills to pay, next week's work, friends to see, hungering aspirations, a myriad of attachments all tend to detract attention from the lessons in casual events.

I thought of this when I visited Capernaum, nestled by the sea of Galilee. It was there that Jesus did most of his teaching. To stand within the foundation marking the primitive synagogue close to the quiet waters of Galilee is to feel the impact of the occurrences that took place there many years ago.

Not far away is the grassy slope of the Mount of the Beatitudes, traditional site of the Sermon on the Mount. As I viewed the scene, I visualized the people gathered together, listening to the words spoken long ago.

It must have been a day similar to the one I was experiencing—warm and sunny with the crest of the hill meeting the blue of the sky. As the words were being uttered, some people were probably thinking of other things, distracted by a honey bee or a restless child. None could possibly have comprehended the unforgettable magnitude of that point in time.

Of similar consequence were my thoughts as I visited some of the great temples in Japan with my friend, Sakan Yanagidaira.

Can you imagine, for example, passers-by attaching any significance to a young man, Siddhartha Guatama, meditating beneath a pipal tree at Bodh Gaya in Nepal years ago? From that fortuitous incident came Buddhism. With that in mind I found the temples such as Horyu-ji (Temple of the Way of Learning) and its architectural treasures of some 40 buildings even more awesome.

On 18 March, 628, two Hinokuma brothers, Hamanari and Takenari went fishing in the Sumida. They found a tiny golden statue and returned it to their native village. It received little notice except from the village headman, Haji-No-Nakatomo who recognized the sanctity of the object and enshrined it. That grew into the Samsoji Temple, one of the most famous centers of Kannon worship in Japan.

But what is true then is also true now. There are events in all of our lives which are of little consequence when they happen, but prove to be of significant value later. Do we have some measurement by which to judge the day-to-day importance of our lives? Learn to learn.

Events are linked together to form chains, each event's karma affecting that of the next one's. Perhaps this is best remembered by the oft-repeated legend based on the defeat of England's King Richard III at the Battle of Bosworth Field in 1485. The army opposing him was led by Henry, Earl of Richmond. The battle would determine who would rule England.

The morning of the conflict, Richard sent a groom with his favorite horse to the blacksmith. But, alas, the blacksmith, having shod many of the horses in the king's army, was out of nails. Since the groom could not wait , the smithy fashioned some nails out of a bit of iron bar. Running out of time and nails, the last shoe was secured with only ill-suited nails on hand.

The armies clashed and Richard rode up and down the lines spurring his men on. Halfway through the battle, with Richard galloping toward some retreating soldiers, one of the horse's shoes fell off. The horse fell, throwing the king to the ground. Then the horse ran off.

Richard's men started turning and running, thinking only of saving themselves. Moments later, Henry's soldiers surrounded Richard and the battle was over.

Since that time, these words have symbolized the linkage of events, one to another:

For want of a nail, a shoe was lost,

For want of a shoe, a horse was lost,

For want of a horse, a battle was lost,

For want of a battle, a kingdom was lost,

And all for the want of a horseshoe nail.

Learning to learn is looking behind every event to determine its cause and possible effects on ensuing events. This is not to predict gloom and doom but to determine karma, risks, and the lessons of life. Lessons will be repeated until learned. Then you can progress to the next one.

MYSTIC DIMENSIONS OF HUMAN LIFE

As you learn to learn you will find that life is really an Odyssey of self-discovery. Untaught phenomena and extra-sensory powers beyond explanation begin surfacing; what is accepted in all other forms of life has somehow been obscured by human beings.

Salmon, for instance, are compelled to struggle upstream. Birds migrate with the seasons. How can a pet cat or dog, lost in travel, make its own way back to its owner thousands of miles away? Such cases are well-documented. Now science is recognizing that the human being has an inner guidance system equally profound. Tuning into that enables one to realize the larger unexplained drama of life.

Significant events, simultaneous occurrences, and chance episodes begin to be perceived as deeply meaningful, holistic experiences. No longer viewed as coincidences, an awareness emerges indicating a cosmic force is at work weaving a unique pattern for each life. There are no random happenings, accidents, or isolated incidents. All of them mesh. They all have meanings. This omniscient characteristic of life is termed "synchronicity."

Dr. Carl Jung, an early colleague of Sigmund Freud, was a forerunner in interpreting synchronicity. He defined it as "the perception of meaningful coincidence." All events are surface effects of a holistic reality existing beyond spirit and matter. Your life is constantly being transformed by forces moving you to become what you are designed to become.

You do not have to understand synchronicity. Just know that it is a power, an energy within, that is one of your resources. Learn to learn. Know that if you put a purpose, a worthy objective in your mind, that you will attract events that will support your endeavor.

Decide, for example, that you want to take a safari to Africa.

You're walking along a shopping mall. Suddenly there's a travel agency. In the window is a display promoting travel in Africa. You meet a friend you haven't seen in months. "Did you know," the friend asks, "that I took a safari to Africa?"

Those are the simpler, more obvious, implications of synchronicity. There are far deeper inferences that can have dramatic effects on the course of your life. What we call fate, chance, or freak incidents are now known as synchronicity. The resulting intuitive impulses have played such an influential part in my life that I have learned to respect each one no matter how seemingly insignificant.

I will share just one example.

Years ago there was a period in my life when I was traveling extensively, working with several projects. While at home one day for only a few hours, I received what would be commonly known as a nuisance phone call.

A strange young voice talked to me about getting together to explore a "business opportunity." I needed him about like a mouse needs a cat. But something kept me on the line. That same something caused me to drive 60 miles the next morning, buy the fellow breakfast, and visit with him for three hours. We talked about direct sales and a marketing plan that his rapidly-growing company was using.

On the way home the idea came to me that those same marketing strategies could be used to distribute some products my Dad had been packaging in his basement. With my father and brother, we put the ideas in place. That was the beginning of the Conklin Company, a company that grew to sell hundreds of millions of dollars of products and affect the lives of thousands of people. I have since divested my ownership in the company. But it is still flourishing and growing today.

Imagine the energy that was capsulated in the coincidental meeting! Dr. Jung proclaimed that as a characteristic of synchronicity. He was having dinner in the 1920's with Einstein, who described the energy hidden within the atom. That was a metaphor for Jung. He reasoned that there were the same inert potentials in synchronicity. By searching within, opening the mind, sensing the meaning of every event, there is a significant release of energy. Learn to learn!

It is easy to count the number of acorns that fall from an oak tree. But it is impossible to count the number of oak trees that can come from a single acorn! You have veiled resources of energy within that can be released and multiplied through synchronicity.

BE SENSITIVE TO YOUR INTUITION

How can you plug into the synchronicity in your life to empower you? Develop and trust your intuitive powers. Albert Einstein said, "It is intuition that improves the world—intuition, not intellect, is the 'open sesame' of yourself."

Intuitive thoughts are nimble, fragile, fleeting thoughts—whirling about in the mind. They are not a part of your rational scripts. They may come tip-toeing into your consciousness at unusual times—while you're walking, shopping, or driving a car. You might be wakened by them in the middle of night or jolted out of a period of meditation. Seize them when they appear. Write them down. They are lessons ignited by synchronicity.

Follow up on your hunches, your intuitive impulses, the feelings within pushing or pulling you on unexplored pilgrimages. Examine them closely. There are risks, of course, and failures. But isn't that the way the child within learned in your earliest days?

Learn to learn. Search within. "A life unexamined is not

worth living," advised Socrates. To deny the mystical thought, the mysteries of life, the unexplainable is to shut one off from the magic of miracles, the limitless dimensions of life.

Venture into the unknown regions of your soul. The mystery of life is the romance, the promise, the excitement of being on this planet. There is a voice of the universe. You are immersed in it. Let it in. Hear it. Open your mind to it. Let it guide you, carry you past the boundaries of your self-imposed territory. Let it free you from human bondage. You will be empowered.

Let's review, again, the "lessons of life."

1. You will learn only what you want to learn when you want to learn it.

2. All events, however trivial, are lessons. Even those events labeled as mistakes, failures, or problems are only lessons.

3. All lessons, properly learned, will lead to your spiritual growth.

4. Lessons are gifts of life. A lesson will be repeated until it is learned. When it is learned you can then go on to the next lesson.

5. The answers to all your questions of what you will become rest within. *"Look well into thyself; there is a source which will always spring up if thou wilt always search there."*
   —*Marcus Aurelius.*

6. Learn to learn for that is the pathway to enlightenment and personal empowerment.

FIFTEEN

Choose to Grow

"There is no sleep, no pause, no preservation, but all
things renew, germinate and spring. Why should
we import rags and relics into the new hour?"
—*Ralph Waldo Emerson*

NINETEEN-YEAR-OLD SCOTT BURGLARIZED AND DID DRUGS. He
was apprehended. The court assigned him to Nexus, our therapeutic
community for young felons, instead of prison.

Scott came in street-smart and con, telling you what he
thought you wanted to hear. Then the therapists and his peers started peeling off veneers of defiance and hostility. The story surfaced
of a childhood devoid of love. Scott was the object of torment and
abuse by his mother and two brothers.

Scott had an agile mind and a staunch spirit. He made
splendid progress, emerging, in fact, as somewhat of a leader. When
he was ready to step into a fresh role in society, an excellent job
opportunity was arranged for him.

The evening before he was to start the new job, Scott asked
me, "I'm scared. I'm really scared. What if I'm not ready? What will
people think of me? Can I handle it?"

"Of course you're scared, Scotty," I said. "It's scary to become
someone other than what you have been. Even if what you have
been has brought you nothing but misery. What lies ahead? The
unknown. But certainly a life better than what you've known."

We talked. "Deal with this," I suggested, "and you can handle just about any situation that comes along. That's growth. It's also the hurdle of growth. Sometimes frightening."

Diane would agree. She worked with us, training corporate facilitators in the use of our programs.

Diane, 24, was tall, lithe, athletic, and excelled in outdoor activities and sports. "I'm leaving," she told me one day. "I've found what I've always dreamed of doing. I'm going to a youth facility in the mountains on the west coast. There I will coach and teach personal development and physical fitness."

"I imagine you're excited," I said.

"Actually I'm frightened," she replied. "This is what I've wanted to do since I was a little girl. It's been a dream, something wonderful to look forward to. Now that it's here, what if it isn't everything I have hoped it would be? What will I do with my life? It will be empty."

No it won't, Diane. For every door that closes another opens, the embers of your soul will still glow and keep life warm and exciting—and growing. For that's the nature of all life—growth. The human spirit was born to grow and stretch as the flower breaks through the ground and reaches for the sun.

So that is the eighth assignment for personal empowerment: "Reach for the sun!" Grow. Stretch. Work toward becoming what you're capable of becoming. All life is either growing or dying, one of the two. Choose to live. Choose to grow.

As Diane and Scott discovered, there can be anxiety about that. Growth means leaving where you are and not coming back. Newness, change, transition can be interesting as long as you have the option of coming back to where you were. If you live in Tokyo and go to London, that can be a jolly fling. You'll be going back home to Tokyo. But what if you can't go back to Tokyo? What if home doesn't exist? That can be frightening.

Think about that. Because you're always changing. You can't go back home. Home doesn't exist. You can't bring back yesterday.

WHAT HAPPENED TO BLACKSMITHS?

About the same thing that happened to men's garters, ice boxes, silent movies, party-line telephones, and women's corsets. They vanished because of change.

Change is a condition of life. Regardless of how pleasurable you found the past, it is gone. Your life is the future. You will be a part of building a fresh tomorrow. There are untried adventures and unlimited opportunities waiting. But they can only be experienced by change. If you are doing things the same way that you did in the past, you will be getting the same results. There are always greater opportunities waiting for you, but only if you are willing to try new ideas and techniques.

Practice change every day. Go to work by a different route. Strike up a conversation with a stranger. Check out a new recipe.

Look for better ways to do your job. Make each day an adventure. Hang on to what works; let go of the old and go for the new. Always be changing, even if only slightly. It is the secret of growth.

The story is told of the Japanese monk who was visiting his Master. The Master started pouring tea in the pupil's cup. When the cup was filled the Master kept pouring. Tea overflowed.

"Stop pouring," said the pupil. "Why do you keep pouring when you see the cup is full?"

"Your mind is like that cup," replied the Master. "Before it can hold more it must first be emptied."

Change empties the mind of the old and makes room for the new. Nature manages the universe in this manner. Without fires to burn out the old woods, new trees and brush would never be nourished by the earth.

So minds need transformation by digesting the past and becoming the food for the future. This is the way humanity progresses and grows. And it is the way the individual grows.

Stretch. Grow. Reach for the sun. Sure, it might mean change, and that takes courage. But courage does not mean being without fear. Courage is tackling all of life's situations, head on, in spite of fear.

Fear can ignite personal growth. "Do the thing you fear the most," is often suggested as an antidote to fear.

Fear can drive you to a higher power. Deep within you is a spirit, a strength, a resource that you may never have been aware existed. Fear may very well bring it to the surface. That's growth. And growth is self-empowering.

"The only thing we have to fear is fear itself!"

Words like those were the artistry of the Franklin Roosevelt speeches that lifted a nation's spirit that had been frayed by depression and war.

What could have been his greatest oration, however, was never delivered. It was to be a Jefferson Day address on April 13, 1945. President Roosevelt had recently returned from Yalta and a conference with Stalin and Churchill. Plans were seeded for the Allied victory and the international gathering in San Francisco to draw up the charter for the United Nations.

Wednesday evening, April 11, Roosevelt finalized his draft of the Jefferson Day address.

The next day, the President was going over some official

papers when he slumped forward, unconscious, at his desk. The rich melodic voice was silenced forever.

If he had lived to speak the next day, the nation would have heard that doubts and fears must be conquered, and that hope must be preserved for a peaceful, happier life for all people throughout the world.

These would have been the final words: "The only limit to our realization of tomorrow will be our doubts of today."

How unfortunate that the sentence was not flung out to be better known.

The only limit to the realization of tomorrow's dreams are the doubts hung on to today.

In the ancient Chinese book of wisdom, I Ching, is the quotation: "All the suffering of mankind is produced by attachment to a previous condition of existence."

What are the "doubts that limit our realization of tomorrow," the "attachment to a previous condition" that causes suffering? It could be like the people in Donner Pass.

GET OUT OF DONNER PASS

In October of 1846, a group of 87 emigrants going to California became trapped by snow. Known as the Donner Party, named for its two Donner families, their fate in the Sierra Nevada is remembered as Donner Pass. Sealed in by heavy snow, their supplies were soon exhausted. After 40 days, half had died of starvation and sickness.

Then two of the men set out to the nearest village. It was, they found, within walking distance. They made it easily and returned with a rescue party to lead the survivors to safety.

Why did they wait 40 days, facing starvation and the risk of death, to leave the site? Why didn't someone venture out before then? It was because they did not want to leave their possessions behind. They grew weak and exhausted attempting to get their wagons and supplies out of the imbedded canyon.

Before you judge those settlers too harshly, imagine, for a moment, that you could be mired in your own Donner Pass. You might be dragging a load of baggage that has your life in a rut.

The further along in life you go, the more baggage and burdens you accumulate. Possessions, obligations, relationships, habits, and routines keep piling up. Each day is a strain to haul the heavy loads along.

You have the feeling that you must get away from it all. The world is closing in on you and there's no way out. You tell yourself that there has got to be more to life than what you are experiencing.

There is! And you can create it! You have been empowered to get far more from life than what you have now. Be willing to let go of the past, take charge of your life and free yourself to create your future. Decide what you want from life.

You have within you the most magnificent mechanism in the universe—your mind. The miraculous powers of the subconscious have never been fully realized by humanity. It is the guiding force that determines your destiny; it will attract and support whatever it is you want. The subconscious mind is always willing to obey the conscious mind. Identify what you want and your subconscious mind will help you get it.

Decide what you want from life. That becomes your vision. Clear your mind of all the garbage and junk that's holding you back. Get clear on your vision. Then focus on it. Don't worry about how you will achieve your vision. Your subconscious will guide you. The process will evolve.

The moment you get clear on what you want then the vision, the dream, will follow. Hold your vision in focus and your inner energies will become mobilized to achieve your desire.

How do you see yourself? Are you in Donner Pass? Do you picture yourself trapped in a job, a set of responsibilities, limitations, obligations and problems from which there is no escape, no freedom? Know that all the conditions you view as narrowing are the very doorways by which you can become free. The promotions that you don't get and the hoped-for success that appears so elusive are all spawning beds for personal growth.

From the problems of those you love that fall as burdens on your heart come the opportunities to give, help, and understand.

From your loneliness and despair come the challenge of looking within and discovering new veins of character, richer emotions, and alternative interests.

From those who criticize, ignore, and mistreat you come the ability to rise above self-pity and gain new strongholds of self-sufficiency.

Because of the love and appreciation you sometimes sense you lack, you can acquire the capacity to love without being loved.

GROW BEYOND LEARNING

Growth is often confused with learning, the cybernation of knowledge, or the enhancement of a skill. One can spend a lifetime absorbing knowledge or mastering a physical craft and still lack maturity and growth. There is an expression for that originating from "The Admirable Crichton." That was a label put on a remarkable young man by one of his biographers. The expression is now used to define a person of a wasted life.

James Crichton was born in 1560 in Scotland. He was probably one of the greatest prodigies who ever lived. At thirteen he was given a college degree of Bachelor of Arts. At seventeen, he was Master of Arts. Within two years he was known throughout Europe as a human encyclopedia, having an amazing command of facts about everything.

He challenged any person to a test of knowledge in any field in open forum. He claimed he could answer any question about anything.

He spoke ten languages fluently. He sang, he painted, he was a sportsman—in short, he did just about anything with exceptional skill which required mental or physical agility.

In his early twenties Crichton was employed to tutor a prince. At twenty-two the Admirable Crichton met death at the hands of the prince, who was in a drunken stupor.

Although it was a tragic end to such an array of fine talent, the world felt little loss. Those who documented his brief life felt that there would have been little difference had he lived to be one hundred.

Crichton was like a giant filing cabinet. A variety of information was digested and filed away but was never applied to any useful purpose. He originated nothing; he worked at nothing; he served no one.

His mind was little more than a remarkable container which was on public display.

Learn, yes, but exert the most enriching learning effort discovering who you are, liking who you are, indeed, loving who you are.

Pearl Buck, American novelist, Nobel and Pulitzer prize winner wrote, "Love dies only when growth stops."

Loving yourself will mount only as you continue to grow. So, reach for the sun, the inner light. Work toward wholeness, know the dimensions of your emotions, the peace and purpose of your spirituality, the depth of your soul. Look within.

GROWTH FROM ADVERSITY

I once planted four Russian olive trees in my back yard. Three did very well, but a fourth, planted too close to my trash burner, became stunted, wilted, and sickly from the heat and smoke of burning rubbish. Somehow it hung on to life and with some watering and fertilizer it survived. Four years later, it was the tallest, fullest, most stately of the four trees. Adversity had strengthened its growth.

In studying the lives of many of the noblest or the famed, there seems to be a common characteristic. They traveled a rocky road, weathered storms of hardship, sickness, and reversal, coming from further back than most, to win the race of expressing their inner greatness. But they persisted, grew, never yielding from becoming what they were destined to become.

That's growth, personal growth toughened by adversity and self-reliance. You can see it in a pine seedling struggling for moisture in a few grains of dirt on a stony mountain side. Does it give up? No! Everyday it strives for nourishment, for born within is the need to grow, to fulfill its life's purpose.

Or a young bird falls from the nest. Those fragile, untaught wings flap instinctively as it scoots for the protection of a bush. Food or warmth is unimportant; this life must fly to survive!

There is a lesson there. For people to untangle the mysteries of the possibilities within them may require facing a stone wall, a barrier, a severe setback—mental or physical. Being bludgeoned and battered by life, having to dig deep to survive, may be the very spawning bed of growth. It is not the way one would choose to grow but it is, indeed, growth.

With growth comes periods of emptiness, voids, that may be distressing, painful, or depressing. But they are necessary for the energy of the soul to exert itself and regenerate growth. The old leaves are dropped to make room for spring's new growth. These pauses in the spiritual journey are the interludes when you sense the discords in life's music and search for the right notes to restore harmony and loveliness to the sounds of your senses.

To grow, hold a mirror to your life. Face it, study it; see its distortions, its sometimes awkwardness and lack of luster. You grow by immersing deeply into life, not running from it or trying to put it behind you as fast as possible. Reach out for life, pull it close to you, embrace it; let it squirm and kick and sometimes fight back. Let it slug you where it hurts worst but don't let it become your enemy or you its victim. As you hold it near to your heart and feel its warmth, you will know all of its rebellion and turmoil is only its striving to be loved. Grow. For love dies only when growth stops.

COMMIT TO GROWTH

Now I have another true story for you. We once owned a home on 12 wooded acres. On the drive approaching the house was an old oak tree that had been hit by lightning and torn apart by windstorms—really just a third of a tree was standing. But it wouldn't stop growing; every spring its stubby branches broke out with a green greeting of leaves.

The fellow who cared for my property and trees wanted to cut it down, claiming that it was ugly—a weed among the roses. But to me it was inspiring, a magnificent testimonial to the energy of growth. Every day I would pass it, revere it, and be reminded that here was life, buffeted and bruised, but still growing empowered rather than weakened by adversity. It was, in fact, committed to growth.

That's a requisite to growth. Commitment.

I am sure that a green apple is very contented just being a green apple. But, alas! As long as it stays attached to a tree branch it must keep working to grow into a ripe red apple. The only way it can possibly remain a green apple is to fall off the tree. Even then it would be short-lived as a green apple because it would gradually waste away.

The same is true of the milkweed seed. The delight of its existence is bursting from its pod and being carried aloft by the silky floss that serves as its very own airline. Airborne, it floats about, freeloading on the lacy puff that lets the breeze decide the adventure of the day. But then the air quiets. The seed settles to the ground. There it becomes captured by the earth where it must start toiling to grow into pale green leaves and purplish flowers. The seed can no longer drift about, just contented as a seed. When held in place by the earth it is committed. It must grow. It has no choice.

The human being is not much different from the green apple or milkweed seed. Where there is no attachment, no commitment, there is no growth. But once an individual is held in place, dedicated by choice or necessity to face every problem, all challenges, the highs and lows of each day, then growth is inevitable.

And, so, the human spirit was born to stretch and grow as the flower breaks through the ground and reaches for the sun. That is the eighth assignment in the quest for self-empowerment. Reach for the sun.

Henry Wadsworth Longfellow must surely have felt some nuances of these thoughts as he wrote his "Psalm of Life" which he said was "a voice from my inmost heart, at a time when I was rallying from depression."

Tell me not, in mournful numbers,
Life is but an empty dream!
For the soul is dead that slumbers,
And things are not what they seem.

Life is real! Life is earnest!
And the grave is not its goal;
Dust thou art, to dust returnest,
Was not spoken of the soul.

Not enjoyment, and not sorrow,
Is our destined end or way;
But to act, that each tomorrow
Find us farther than today.

Say "Yes" to Life

Life is real! Life is earnest! Say "Yes" to it. Far too much of life is cut short by "no" rather than "yes." A heart full of despairs, failures, loneliness, and boredom is caused by saying "no" instead of "yes." But that's the way you were taught.

From the time of your first wobbling steps, "no" was used to curb the childish wildness, not just a few "noes," but thousands. A big heap more "noes" than "yeses" soaked into your sponge-like subconscious only to be dribbled out slowly during your adult span along with "can't," "don't," "mustn't" and "stop it!" Even the Ten Commandments are eight "shall nots" and only two "shalls." There are over 1,300 "noes" and only four "yeses" in the Bible.

Human beings and the universe are powered by streams of energy. Thought is an energy. Healing is an energy. Love is an energy. Life, itself, is energy. You cause those energies to flow through you by "yes." You shut them off by "no." Those who are cutting themselves away from these natural forces by their "noes" are like Westchester, a Chicago suburb. For seven years this chagrined community experienced a water shortage. Then somebody discovered that the three main valves governing its water supply had never been fully turned on!

Open the channels of your thoughts so that life can flow through you, unobstructed by old barriers.

Get yourself turned on by saying "yes"! Say "yes" to untried experiences! Say "yes" to helping others! Say "yes" to unexplored pathways! Say "yes" to breaking old habits.

Say "yes" to your emotions, needs, and wants. Say "yes" to a different way of relating to a friend or marriage partner. Go out for breakfast. Play checkers. Read a book together. Have hot dogs in the park.

Say "yes" to the quiet moments alone. Spin off from the humdrum. Think. Dream. Rest. Break away from the obsession that you must be doing something every waking minute.

This does not imply that you should say "yes" to those who want your possessions or want to take advantage of you. It means saying "yes" to yourself and life.

Say "yes" to your wonder and magnificence. Stop thinking that incredible success and happiness belongs to a favored few. The world is for you, not against you, right now, today! Life is not what is happening some day. The only life that you can know is today, this hour, this minute. Say "yes" to the moment! This day can be twice as joyous as yesterday, if you believe it. You choose the results of your life by choosing your thoughts.

Say "yes" to those inner urges, the sleeping dreams and the timid hopes. Your instincts are crying out desperately for you to say "yes" to the greatness and the limitless potential within you.

You don't express your own splendor by looking for things wrong or waiting. Nor do you do it by defending and protecting the way you are or the rituals and habits of your life. Change, admittedly, can be risky. It means leaving where you are and not coming back. You must step out of the comfort zone and be uncomfortable. That requires mental and physical stamina, courage, and even some distress. It's easier to say "no" to that than "yes." But those "noes" are ways of simply repeating what the past has been. Saying "yes" opens up all sorts of possibilities.

SAY "YES" TO YOUR CREATIVITY

Be like Miss Scheherazade in The Arabian Nights. King Shahriar married one wife after another simply to cut off their heads. Scheherazade was forced to become his wife. She then captured his fancy by telling a different story every night for one thousand and one nights. He kept postponing her killing to see what the next story was going to be.

After three years, she won the king's love and kingdom!

Among her stories was Aladdin and his magic lamp. It was a legacy left for all. It is the gift of creativity. You have it within you. It is so powerful and limitless that its wonder is almost beyond comprehension.

The human imagination is the greatest untapped resource in the world. Ideas, seeded and nourished, can shape abundance and distinction for any who care to invest the effort.

You may feel you are not a creative person. That is not true. All have creative ability.

Education is no factor in creative talent except, at times, to suppress creativity. One survey showed that the more education people have, the less likely they are to be inventive.

Past training has little effect on creativity. The telegraph was worked out by Morse, a professional portrait painter. Robert Fuller, an artist, invented the steamboat. One of the great composers of American music, Irving Berlin, was a waiter who never learned to play the piano, except by ear and in F sharp.

Creativity has little relationship to age. Alexander the Great was a creative genius in many ways other than military. He conquered Persia at the age of 25. Grandma Moses started painting when she was 70. Benjamin Franklin was at his creative best when he was past 80. The first time George Bernard Shaw won a Nobel Prize he was 70. He was still going strong in his 90s.

In fact, creating seems to strengthen and prolong life. The Council on Aging reports that people live longer who are motivated to create.

That force of motivation seems to be the fountain from which creativity flows. For ideas do not occur by accident or impulse. They grow from a deliberate quest planted in the mind and then fueled by effort.

Creativity is a process more than a revelation. It is triggered by a question. Feeding a question to your imagination is more productive than pushing the keys on a computer. You will infallibly get a variety of possibilities. They will continue to flow if you continue to keep an open mind.

The question can be in the form of problems. That is why problems are opportunities. They stimulate creativity. Most of what is known today as progress started first as a problem and was transformed into an idea.

Do you have problems or limitations? Program them into your imagination. Hold them there. Don't let them go until they burst into possibilities. Then, write them down and put them to work. The more you practice this, the better you will become.

Creativity is like any other developed talent. You use it or lose it. What a precious gift it is to lose, this Aladdin's lamp, that can truly light up your life!

The planet is flourishing with creativity and growth. And, remember? You are a microcosm of the planet. So, say "yes" to your creativity. Stretch. Reach. Grow. Love dies only when growth stops.

SAY "YES" TO YOUR PURPOSE

We are here to express God, to love, to serve, to glorify God's dream for life. There is no other reason, no other meaning greater than that.

There is a divine purpose for your life. Say "yes!" to that purpose. Make it your mission, your passion; let it be merged with your spiritual quest. Life does not sort out purposes as large or small. No matter whether you are sorting papers, raising rice, caring for the sick, tending a home or building a shrine, they are all purposes and worthy of your devotion. Celebrating the sunrise of each day by exerting your energy, your grace, your humility towards your purpose adds splendor to each of life's moments. Welcome the weariness that such activity brings. Be concerned only when that is lacking.

I pray that the words and ideas you and I have shared have nourished your empowerment that you may better reflect God's dream for you. It was Oliver Wendell Holmes who said, "Alas, for those who never sing but die with all their music in them."

So my wish is that you have grown and continue to grow— to express the greatness within you. For love dies only when growth stops.

It is time now that we part. Reluctantly, I might add. For my heart and mind are telling me to keep on writing. A long-time friend, Jesse Lair, who authored several best sellers, once told me, "You never get through writing a book. You finally reach a point when you just let it go."

So I have reached the time when I know I must just "let it go."

I hope we can meet again for sharing words and ideas. That might be in a sort of ethereal sense. Your God-child and my God-child may be in touch from time to time.

But, wait a moment! How could I forget?

Of course they will be in touch. For they are, in truth, one.

So be it.

God bless you!

Credits

Reference is made in this book to other works by Robert Conklin. The POSITIVE MIND ALBUM is a five hour audio cassette enrichment course. ADVENTURES IN ATTITUDES and LIFEPOWER are thirty hour personal development programs. Information about these three programs may be obtained from:

Carlson Learning Company
Carlson Parkway
P.O. Box 59159
Minneapolis, MN 55459
(612) 449-2882